MARCUS ANTEBI
THE FOUNDER OF JUICE PRESS

THE goodsugar DIET™

LOSE WEIGHT
BURN FAT
BOOST IMMUNITY
AND EXPAND
YOUR MIND

Edited by John Geib, Jill Goldhand, and Rachel Weber

> Dear
> This book have been done without you— all the best
> Marcus A.

The goodsugar Diet™

Lose Weight
Burn Fat
Boost Immunity
And Expand Your Mind

Copyright 2020 by Marcus Antebi. All rights reserved. Printed in the United States of America. No part of this book may be used or reproduced in any manner whatsoever without written permission. For information please contact goodsugar™ at info@goodsugar.life

Library of Congress Cataloging-in-Publication Data has been applied for.
ISBN: 978-1-7354707-7-1

For additional support pages for this program:
www.goodsugardiet.com

Listen to: www.goodsugarpodcast.com

Table of Contents

Foreword 1

Part 1: Orientation 3

1. Why I Can Help You 3
2. Who This Book Is For and How to Use It 5
3. Purpose and Structure of This Book 9
4. The Secret to Self-Help 15
5. Maintaining Healthy Dietary Patterns Is a Big Step Towards Self-Mastery 18
6. You're a Pig! 22
7. Starting a New Diet Creates Hope 27
8. Get Excited About Starting Your Journey 31
9. This Book Will Help You—I Guarantee It 34
10. What Kind of Eater Are You? 36
11. What Is Self-Improvement? 39
12. We Must Be Honest With Ourselves 42
13. This Is a Challenging, Worthwhile Journey You Will Succeed At 44
14. Distraction and Lack of Good Habits 45
15. Practice, Not Perfection 46

Part 2: The Primary Work 47

16. Create a Journal and Always Write in It 47
17. Who Else Journaled Throughout History? You're Not a Dweeb for Writing 51
18. Important Writing Assignments 52
19. The Power of the Task List 53

20.	The Importance of Saying the Right Words and Taking the Right Actions	54
21.	Celebrate the Beginning of This New Journey	56
22.	Your Dietary Changes Will Help Stop War and Starvation	58
23.	Comparing Food Addiction to Other Common Addictions	60
24.	Expand Your Consciousness—Everyone's Doing It	61
25.	Become Fully Aware of Your Childhood Experiences—Stop Denying	62
26.	Consciousness Expanding Lifestyle Practices	63
27.	The Pursuit of Mental Health Is the Pursuit of Consciousness	64
28.	Move Past Traumatic Experiences by Writing About Them	65

Part 3: The Psychology Work **69**

29.	Losing Weight is Not Just for Vanity—It's for Our Peace of Mind	69
30.	The Psychological Program	72
31.	Smash Denial: Admit That You Have a Problem	73
32.	Behavior Patterns Trigger Poor Dietary Choices	77
33.	The Relationship Between Physical Exercise and Happiness	80
34.	Stop Saying Unkind Things to Yourself	81
35.	About Childhood Trauma	85
36.	Addressing Childhood Trauma and Emotional Issues	88

37.	Identify Difficult Emotional Checkpoints That Lead to Negative Behavior...............	91
38.	Feel Your Feelings	92
39.	Bodily Processing of Emotions	99
40.	Repressing Emotions Can Make Us Physically and Emotionally Sick..........	101
41.	Therapy Is Important	103
42.	A Story Illustration	106
43.	Peoples' Motivations for Going on Diets	108
44.	The Error of Seeking Dietary Advice	109
45.	Mealtimes and Misconceptions..........	110
46.	Food Cravings	112
47.	Sweet Tooth.........................	114
48.	What the Heck Are We Really Craving?.....	117
49.	How to See the Supermarket Experience ...	120
50.	Cravings and Emotional Food Attachments .	121

Part 4: The Dietary Change Work **125**

51.	Eliminate Processed Food From Your Diet ..	125
52.	Toxic Food Processing.................	128
53.	Diet Plan Considerations	138
54.	Food Disorder Syndromes..............	140
55.	Addictive Food Types..................	142
56.	Supermarket Food Issues	143
57.	Nutrition: An Overview	146
58.	What Is Food?	147
59.	Plant-Based: The Optimal Diet for Humans..	148
60.	Fear of Not Getting Enough Protein in Your Diet............................	150
61.	Change Your Dietary Perspective	153

62.	Food Is Fuel, Not Medicine	155
63.	What Is Not Food?	156
64.	Understand Nutritional Needs and Principles: Misconceptions Regarding Nutrition	157
65.	Calories	158
66.	Protein	162
67.	Carbohydrates	163
68.	Fat	164
69.	Vitamins and Minerals	165
70.	Seasonal Foods	168
71.	You Are What You Eat—Eats	169
72.	Consider Vegetarianism	170
73.	The Primary Food Sources: Humans Versus Other Animals	171
74.	The Plant-Based Diet	171
75.	Good Plant Foods and Where to Find Them	175
76.	I Am Obsessed With Fruits, Vegetables, Nuts, Sprouts, and Seeds	176
77.	Water and Hydration	178
78.	Fall in Love With Salad	183
79.	Fall in Love With Juices and Smoothies	187
80.	Development in Human Diet Patterns	190
81.	Cow's Milk and Chicken Eggs	191
82.	Don't Let Pious Vegans Judge You	195
83.	Ethical Considerations	199
84.	Alcohol, Tobacco, Inhaling Smoke From Cannabis, and Other Drugs	201
85.	What About Coffee?	202
86.	Cacao (Chocolate) and Maca	208
87.	Other Hippie Weirdo Products	208
88.	USDA Organic Certified Produce	209

Part 5: Advanced Work Into Action............ 213

- 89. Vital Force 213
- 90. Getting Rid of Food Contraband 214
- 91. Late Night Safety Measures to Protect Against Emotional Eating................ 216
- 92. Set Eating Times for Each Meal. Create Repetition and a Pattern........... 218
- 93. Avoiding Fad Diets..................... 219
- 94. Ancient Ayurvedic and Chinese Medicine Diets................................... 220
- 95. About the Term "Biohack" 222
- 96. Fasting and Juice Cleanses.............. 224
- 97. Intermittent Fasting: Create Longer Periods of Daily Abstinence Before Eating 228
- 98. Details Regarding Fasting Practices 230
- 99. My Experience With Cravings 230
- 100. Exercise More and More, Get It In 231
- 101. The Mindset of Exercise................. 235
- 102. Suggested Exercise Types............... 237
- 103. Walking Is the Most Important Exercise..... 238

Part 6: Essential Mindfulness, Meditation, Prayer, and Service........................ 241

- 104. Relax Before Meals and Focus During Mealtimes............................. 241
- 105. Visualize Your Body as You Want It to Be ... 243
- 106. Meditation: An Introduction 245
- 107. For the Most Distracted People in the World. 246
- 108. Don't Forget Prayer, Even if You're an Atheist.. 247
- 109. Positive and Negative Thoughts 250
- 110. Gratitude 253

111. How to Meditate................................ 257
112. Meditation Is a Long-Term Practice......... 263
113. Apology Accepted 264
114. Helping Others and Being of Service........ 267

Part 7: Integrating and Incorporating This Program Into Your Life........................ 271

115. Make a Daily Ritual of Returning to Your Shrine to Recommit to Your Recovery...... 271
116. This Program Is a New Power 273
117. Taking Ownership and Dietary Transition.... 274
118. A Final Pitch on Veganism and Avoiding Processed Food........................... 275
119. Food Industry Issues 276
120. Energy of Food........................... 277
121. Abstinence 277
122. Elimination and Irregularity................ 278
123. Dietary Issues and Irregularity 281
124. Suggested Remedies for Irregularity 283
125. Keeping a Scale in the House 284
126. Your Relationship With Food and Lifestyle Choices Moving Forward.................. 285
127. Get Into Therapy 287
128. Bond With Nature........................ 290
129. Sleep Is an Integral Part of Weight Loss and an Overall Sense of Well-Being 293
130. Supplements in General................... 296
131. Probiotic Supplements.................... 297
132. A Glimpse Into My Personal Story......... 298
133. A Cup of Tea............................. 302
134. Therapy and Determination 303

135. Summary and Recap	303
136. My Top 30 Positive Health and Lifestyle Changes/Behaviors	310
137. Maintenance: We Need Daily Tune-Ups	315
138. Confusement	315
139. Self-Acceptance: When You Have It, You Know You Are Getting Well	317
140. Recovering From Mistakes and Relapses	317
141. Inspiration to Continue Getting Better	318
About the Author	321

Acknowledgements

I must acknowledge the teachings of my dear friend and food mentor: Fred Bisci. Without his direction, I would be miles off course.

I want to express my deepest gratitude to my wife Teresa and to my daughter Luna. My love for them has opened my eyes. Of course my daughter Minnie and my wife's children Zaria and Lion are all three treasures of my life.

To my father David, my mother Marilyn and sister Raquel: We have all been on this long and strange journey together. I love you and I wish that you three more than all people find something helpful in my writing. I wish you health and freedom from suffering.

Foreword

"Diet": A noun, a verb, or a way of life? We are engulfed with the pressures of life, our families, friends, work, play, politics, and cosmic questions we fall back on when truly on the spot. But where does our health fit in? "Health": This is, in fact, the key to all of the answers, since our physical well-being fashions our emotional well-being, attitudes, and approaches. Health is our ticket for success and self-esteem.

Transforming the idea and target of health into real action is yet another critical question. There are many options, as there are many different flavors of people. Now, the true question is, how does one get motivated to be healthy? If reaching a level of human performance that can approach, touch, and even grab a wild dream has appeal, then reading The goodsugar Diet™ by Marcus Antebi is a worthwhile endeavor. Marcus has already proven to be a successful innovator in health and nutrition through his founding of Juice Press and is now extending his philosophy of living in this book.

Here's what lies ahead. Marcus offers a perspective that will resonate; a message that is conversational, but has the raw physics of power and energy that motivate change. From a medical standpoint, it is a person's "activation for change" that is the first step toward improvement and a more healthy lifestyle.

There are clear tactics to achieve this change outlined in the pages that follow: keeping a journal; creating a "to do" list; introspection and reflecting on your personal history; and simply being nice to yourself. The fuel that impels the reader is the rapid exploration of terrain, the quick starts, bumps and jerks, and the hurdles that define a roller coaster experience through the burgeoning field of healthy eating patterns. This is a holistic maneuver that culminates in a final "aha," where being healthy is realistic, easy, happy and fun.

So, make yourself comfortable and enjoy the ride.

JEFFREY I. MECHANICK, M.D., F.A.C.P., F.A.C.N., E.C.N.U., M.A.C.E.

Professor of Medicine and Medical Director of The Marie-Josee and Henry R. Kravis Center for Clinical Cardiovascular Health at Mount Sinai Heart

Director, Metabolic Support, Division of Endocrinology, Diabetes and Bone Disease, Icahn School of Medicine at Mount Sinai, New York

PART ONE
ORIENTATION

1. Why I Can Help You

My name is Marcus Antebi. I was born in Brooklyn, New York in 1969, and I am grateful because I've had a rich and full life that I plan to continue for the next 50+ years.

I survived 13 years of skydiving and retired with over 2,300 jumps. I survived competitive Muay Thai fighting. I started a juice company called Juice Press in 2010, and when I exited we had 85 stores.

The thing that makes me qualified to write this book is the most noteworthy thing that I've done in my life: I've been clean and sober since 1985 when I overcame my addiction to marijuana. I tried all kinds of drugs, and by the time I was 15 1/2 years old I was done. I went to an inpatient rehabilitation facility for 90 days.

Some thought that inpatient treatment seemed a little bit dramatic for marijuana addiction, but I found it necessary. I'm glad that I requested that level of treatment, and it served to get me on a path of lifetime recovery.

I also became passionate about recovery in the process of growing up watching my father and sister struggle with their weight and the role of food in their lives. Doing so left a painful impression on me—I felt powerless to ease their suffering. I was very close to my father and I spent years trying to understand his childhood and how his trauma was associated with his diet and lifestyle patterns. I believe I developed a complex from my father's problems. I wanted to save my family from their addictions and suffering, but I wasn't able to. So, I am converting all of my pent-up energy, emotions, and knowledge of the subject matter into this project and a number of similar efforts. I find that writing out and organizing information focused on self-help topics is very satisfying and therapeutic to me.

At Juice Press I needed to be a prolific writer of many kinds of self-help and commerce-related documents for customers and team members. Now I'm excited to move on to books.

My mentor is a great man named Fred Bisci. At the time of this writing he is 90 years young and has been 100% raw vegan for approximately 55 years. He had a nutritional practice for many years and has a remarkably deep level of understanding of diet and the human body. I am a devoted vegan myself.

I've been practicing yoga since 1997. More than any other type of physical exercise, practicing yoga has been the thing that has helped me learn how to concentrate and focus; that is something that was always very difficult for me. This focus has helped me keep positive and avoid my tendency towards addiction.

That's essentially my story. I don't have university degrees or formal education; my college education took place on the streets and in the process of being wholeheartedly devoted to living and instructing others in healthy lifestyle practices over a 35-year period.

Writing about health and wellness is something that I have become very passionate about. I stepped down from Juice Press in order to focus primarily on this book and getting this important plan out to you.

My current health and wellness company, goodsugar™, is a platform for helping us improve and maintain our health. I'm not seeking to just sell products. In my life and in my companies, social and environmental responsibility is still of paramount importance. I want to help people get on the right path to a lifestyle that incorporates good physical and mental health, respect for our planet, and service to others.

I sincerely hope that my writing will be encouraging and beneficial to you as you seek to make yourself a better person and our world a better place.

2. Who This Book Is For and How to Use It

This book is for anyone who wants to be truly healthy and happy. It will offer you many weight loss tips, and some of those tips will help you to lose weight fairly quickly. What it will not offer you is a quick fad diet enabling you to lose a few pounds over a weekend. Instead, this book will encourage you to make all-encompassing lifestyle changes. Such changes will enable you to not only lose weight, but to keep the weight off, change your body chemistry for the better, and engage in a positive journey to attain excellent mental, physical, and emotional health and wellness.

Toxic diets and bad eating habits are prevalent in all countries, regardless of the races, creeds, and religions practiced by those countries' inhabitants. The United States can no longer take the National Blue Ribbon Award for "Country With The Worst Diet." Worldwide, we have strayed far away from what is ideal for us, while what is ideal for us is still debated.

This problem emerged around the same time that kingdoms with large cities did. People shifted to singular, skyward-facing gods instead of regarding earthly locations and earthly abundance as sacred. We slowly converted from hunter-gatherers who had deep connections with all aspects of the land to large populations of malnourished dependents.

From this emerged large-scale agriculture, large-scale warfare, pandemics, superstition, science, modern-day commerce, the FDA, and the place where humanity is now with rampant obesity and food-related illnesses!

Our problems with food today are interwoven with mistakes passed on from generation to generation over a long period of time. But you can help change this situation for the better!

As individuals like you become more aware and positively shift your eating patterns, you are changing the entire world. This is how consciousness works: Your awareness and consciousness become part of a collective consciousness.

The fundamental components of existence are air, water, **FOOD**, shelter, warmth, human contact, safety, habits and routines, dignity, love, enjoyment, stillness, and connection with the cosmos and divine consciousness. Today, most people are divorced from the third most fundamental component of their existence, FOOD.

This book is about food. However, all of our absolute necessities are bound together by the same thread. The thread is mechanically linked to the laws of the Universe. Whether you read this as a spiritual statement or as an intellectual one (as I intended it to be) does not matter as long as you receive the message.

I have learned that the correct path to relearning food and dietary patterns must be a holistic, all-encompassing one that entails surrender. It's necessary to surrender yourself in order to master yourself. Surrender to your healing. Surrender to pain. Surrender to your amazing power to recover and grow. Surrender to compassionate words. Surrender and lead yourself toward self-realization right now! Surrendering may be a gradual process that takes time, or you may be able to do so in an instant—it could take one second or it could take your entire life.

There's absolutely nothing better that you could be doing than living your life in the best way possible right now. If you can't do that, it may be that you're stuck in something that's difficult to deal with. We all get stuck. Some more so than others. But the ones who are the most stuck then recover to become some of the most amazing healers and creators of all time.

Let's not be sad and let's not feel alone. We are not alone. Plus, it seems that every single human that ever existed struggled. There's nothing wrong with you and there's nothing wrong with me. We are just working on things and figuring sh*t out. So take a deep breath and thank someone or something that you love that we are here and that we will be for a long enough time.

Do you really need anyone's help in dealing with food and dietary issues? The answer is almost certainly yes. Maybe you have 200 pounds to lose, or maybe just three to five pounds of excess weight that keeps you from being totally in love with your body. We're all on a similar journey to better health in general and weight control in particular, and we can all benefit from the input of others to some degree.

Having spent more than a decade in the health and wellness food industry, I have determined who can benefit most from this particular book. This book is best suited for people whose diets have made them feel like they've "hit bottom"—people who are more than ready to make critical lifestyle changes.

I don't offer cheats, fast tips, or shortcuts. **If you've been a consumer of diet products, then you realize that eventually all of those things fail us.**

At this point, hopefully, you are ready to do the repair work that's both necessary and effective. You will have to take your own journey to understand your all-encompassing relationship with food and with all of the substances that you put into your body.

If you're ready to do this work, understand that it will take time. But with time, you will gain greater self-awareness, more depth, healing, and you will grow to feel good about your entire life. When your diet is part of an all-encompassing lifestyle change, you will reach more of your overall goals. You will be on your path to a happy and healthy life.

There's quite a bit of content in this book. Each section is numbered, and the various sections can be read in any order over any amount of time. I recommend that you take this book with you everywhere you go and read from it constantly. Even if all you can handle is one minute at a time or half a section at a time, keep the book with you. Keep it by your bedside. Randomly open it to any page at any time and read; it is all useful, helpful and life-affirming.

During the early years of my recovery, I had many books similar to this. I kept them next to my bedside and in my backpack. I'd continually read portions of them at different times, and I gleaned through the various books until their messages sank in.

Generally speaking, it's very difficult for a person who is confused about their overall life and the circumstances around them to take in new things. If you're in such a situation, you'll find it helpful to surround yourself with things that help you learn. This book will help you learn, so keep it close.

3. Purpose and Structure of This Book

The purpose of this book is to help anyone interested in weight loss, weight control and good health make a number of dietary changes for the better. The first such change is to abstain from processed foods. Next, I want to help readers make all of the other tweaks to diet and overall lifestyle that I know will cause them to function and feel better: Functioning and feeling better are critical in sustaining long term weight and health goals. Finally, my goal is to help readers look deeper into their emotions and thought patterns in order to develop a greater sense of peace. I am hoping to help you find your way back to your path of self-realization. The first step is to change the patterns in our lives that lead to suffering and distraction.

I have divided this book into seven parts: (1) Orientation; (2) The Primary Work; (3) The Psychology Work; (4) The Dietary Change Work; (5) Advanced Work Into Action; (6) Essential Mindfulness, Meditation, Prayer, and Service; and (7) Integrating and Incorporating This Program Into Your Life.

Each subpart of the book is numbered as a section (from 1 to 141). The numerical order of these subparts does not necessarily reflect their value in importance from highest to lowest. Each subpart is a critical component of this comprehensive program.

This book was not created as a highly commercialized diet program with unrealistic or impossible promises of success. It's not at all along the same lines as the old Thigh Master® TV commercials. Thigh Master® was much easier than anything I know of in the health industry.

This program is a true self-help guide. The emphasis is on *self*, meaning that you have to do all of the work. This program has no contraptions, no 14-day promises, and no miracle pills. Only your correct decisions and efforts over the long term will deliver lasting results for you.

Having said that, I must be truthful and say that almost any popularized diet that requires that you abstain from processed food, no matter how ineffective the rest of the program may be, will work to help you lose weight and feel better. While that may be enough for some. But many studies and my experience observing others have shown me that if no other steps are taken, the weight comes right back after a short period of time.

Even diets that seem to be sustainable for a few months or years are not worth the superficial benefit of a tight and toned body if those diets are toxic to our chemistry. They can be toxic because they require that we exaggerate the macronutrients to one degree or another. They may also require that we eat far too much animal protein in particular than what the natural parameters of the human body are set to function best at.

Tightness and good tone may be indicators of only one aspect of health; we can have six-pack abs and still be on a collision course with illness and disease.

This program focuses on all-encompassing lifestyle and diet choices. The program in this book is comprehensive and it will require a great deal of attention, focus and concentration on the things we are about to look at. It will also require time on the reader's part to absorb all of the comprehensive content. It will take longer than "The 7 Minute Abs" program takes, but it will offer a great deal more.

If any person follows this program step by step, they will get better. I know this to be true from my own life experiences as well as from my interactions with others, including extensive consultations with nutritionists and medical doctors.

The website *www.goodsugar.life* will complement this book. It will offer many more suggestions relating to dietary choices and lifestyle practices.

Be patient as you embark on this journey. Make changes at a pace that is suitable to your comfort level. If you're consistent and focused as you do so, you will experience impressive results. Even if you are drowning in your distractions right now, just holding this book and striving to read each page is going to make you better.

There are many things that prevent us from reaching a true emotional and physical bottom regarding our weight loss and negative dietary patterns. Sometimes being fantastically wealthy or being well-off in other ways can make us so comfortable that we don't ever really hit an emotional bottom. We get close, but we've got enough distractions around us to keep us from really hitting that bottom and saying, "I'm done, I'm fed up, I've got to do something now!" And sometimes even when we hit bottom we do not know what to do next. We might drift for a while at the bottom and then resume our old bad habits.

We may have enablers in our lives who make it really easy for us to continue our unhealthy behavior. Perhaps they cook for us a certain way, or maybe they keep the house filled with junk food. If you haven't reached the bottom, it's going to be difficult for you to breeze through this comprehensive program. The reason this is so is that the program requires long-term concentration and focus, dedication, motivation, character development, personal growth, and building higher levels of self-esteem.

If you have resistance to being uncomfortable, as most of us do, then making a change, getting up, doing the necessary work, and reading a book like this will require a push from someone like me. I will push you gently. Please allow me to be your guide. You can do everything in this book, and you will!

This book could easily be 5,000 pages long because there's always something helpful pertaining to weight loss, general health, self-improvement, and being happy that could be added. The book isn't a novel with stories of lovers rolling around on the beach. There's no intriguing mystery here, and there's no surprising, twisted ending. This book consists of straightforward direction. It condenses and summarizes my lifelong experiences in health and wellness, dietary and otherwise, with a focus on things that have worked for myself and countless others.

You will find this book to be quite different from most books that speak of diet and nutrition. This is so because I've found it necessary to cover quite a number of things and to focus on three issues in particular.

One issue is the shortcomings of certain popular diet programs. Another is the necessity of incorporating all-encompassing holistic lifestyle practices into weight control and health improvement efforts. The third issue pertains to the use of sound psychological and metaphysical principles when approaching lifestyle changes of any kind.

There's certainly a lot of content in this program to unpack and assimilate. This program was not designed to deliver mind-blowing results in 14 days. Making substantial improvements in diet and lifestyle takes time and continuous effort. Popular diets are very successful because of the way that they package their programs. They make users believe that there's an incredibly simple way to lose weight and then live happily ever after, even if the users don't make many changes to their long-term dietary practices and lifestyle patterns.

Psychology is of critical importance in long-term sustainable weight loss, weight control, and healthy living, but some of us are intimidated by books on psychology. This is so for a couple of reasons. At times the material that's covered in those types of books seems pedantic and dry, and as such not particularly interesting to read. And another issue is that the material is sometimes presented in a way that doesn't give readers sufficient guidance on how to apply the valuable insights and principles to their daily lives.

Spiritual books often bring us comfort—they can be inspiring and encouraging. But the subject matter is often not contextual enough for those who wish to apply spiritual principles to their specific dietary needs and struggles. Although spirituality looms large in dietary change efforts, the current pantheon of books about diet and lifestyle do not address such changes to a sufficient enough degree in a spiritual context.

I've needed a book such as this my entire life. I needed it 35 years ago when I was a very uneducated eater intoxicating myself daily with food. Even with the changes I have made, I still need this book today. I wrote this book to give back what I learned in the hope that others will find it useful. I practice all of these principles in my daily life, and I have been sober regarding my eating behaviors for 25 years, and 35 years with regard to drugs and alcohol.

To elaborate a bit on diet plans that sound absurdly simple, they almost never work past the short term. This is the case because they don't specify all of the work that the dieter needs to do. They usually focus almost entirely on food. They almost never address behavior and don't provide steps to deal with deeply-rooted emotions that trigger bad dietary habits. It's unpopular to tell dieters that difficult psychological work on their part is a necessary component of permanent weight loss. For that reason, diet programs that emphasize hard work and sometimes painful introspection don't sell well.

Many, perhaps most people aren't interested in diving deep and getting their weight control problems fixed once and for all, or they are unable to see the connection between psychology and weight loss. Popular diet programs don't often get to the heart of our issues with food. One has to overcome a lifetime of bad habits, developed to anesthetize their pain, in order to create healthy habits around food. We have anxiety, lack of focus, lack of discipline, and lack of knowledge, all of which work against us in weight control and healthy living.

It may seem harsh that I am saying these things right off the bat. But I want to help you. And I know how stubborn we all can be, because I'm the same way. I often go in and out of my own denial. Denial about old and new feelings. Denial about a problem, its cause, and then resistance to doing the work to improve. This kind of work requires a daily pledge, from now until the day we leave the body. We must take an interest in our health improvement and the actions required to achieve it!

Throughout this book, sometimes I'll speak to you with a lot of compassion. Other times I'll present you with disturbing information about you and the things you eat that will probably make you upset. Everybody, including myself, needs a wake-up call when they're doing something that puts them at risk.

I will repeat this over and over again: Many weight loss programs seem simple on the surface. But, again, much more often than not, they don't work. You're usually trained like a circus animal to perform tricks on your body. The methodologies that fad diets employ consist of what are popularly termed "biohacks." These diets work to a degree, but they are not the winning solution to the good health, long-term weight loss, and weight control that you desperately need.

The winning solution consists of the steps outlined in this book. I know this from personal experience. I am asking you to make the program described in this book your top priority for several months. After reading this book in its entirety and making an honest, concerted effort to put its information into practice, keep going back to it. You will find things that you may have missed in earlier readings, and you will find things that are particularly applicable to things going in your life at that point in time as you progress on your journey.

As you do so, not only will you lose weight and keep it off, but your attention span will improve, you will become more focused, and your overall physical and mental health will improve tremendously. The more you hear the invaluable messages presented in this book, the more they will stick.

This book details a comprehensive weight loss and lifestyle improvement program that can be implemented by anyone. This first edition covers quite a bit of ground, addressing a wide variety of interrelated topics. I will make every effort to make whatever stylistic corrections are warranted in future editions. But I am asking you to seriously consider the book's content and make the commitment to do the work.

4. The Secret to Self-Help

There are two epic secrets to improving one's life. One of them is to train yourself to take baby steps in everything that you do in connection with self-help. For example, if a book is really thick and it's promising to teach you how to liberate yourself from pain and suffering, you might keep that book on your shelf for 10 years because its size intimidates you. Think about the irony in that.

A book that promises to relieve us from our suffering sits untouched for years—we would rather suffer than make small efforts toward improvement. Why is that? It's because we are afraid of a shift in reality, or because we don't know how to take the first step and so we become paralyzed, or it may simply be that we never grew out of being lazy. It makes no difference what the causes of inaction are: We need to solve the problem, and the way to solve this problem is to take steps—really, really small steps—and take them every day.

Every time something becomes too big of a step, break it down into smaller steps. Read one page in this book every day. Just one page is all you need, and you'll be drifting into the path of wellness. Not because I am a guru, or that my words are great, but because you are taking action.

The next secret to learning great lessons is to teach them. That is the essence of 12-step recovery, which we can borrow from. The 12th step in recovery is about being of service and helping others. The reason why this is put into action in a self-help program is because if a person is busy trying to show others how to help themselves, they're teaching themself that same lesson. Therefore, anything that you are struggling with, find someone struggling with the same thing to a greater degree, and help them. There is always someone out there who can benefit from your kindness and compassion. (More about this later.)

Back to taking baby steps. If we're having trouble starting an activity that seems too difficult, we're likely not aware of how to break it down into smaller tasks that are easier to accomplish. Maybe we have to break that task down into five or ten smaller steps.

I will use my early experience with meditation as an example. I first thought that meditation was a waste of time because I could not connect with the universe and creation and become fully enlightened the first time I tried it. I could not approach meditation because I could not imagine myself sitting and wrestling with boredom for an hour. The idea of meditation seemed pointless because I did not feel any benefits right from the start. Instead of relaxing me, it made me more stressed out than before.

But then I realized that if I approached meditation the way I approached building a retail store—incrementally, step-by-step—I could accomplish something. In building, I was patient with the process. Each day we would finish a little bit more and then move on to the next thing. We couldn't start electrical work until we framed the walls. We couldn't build a cabinet until the floor was complete.

I can approach meditation in the same manner. I can sit for two minutes and say, "I am meditating," over and over again. I can declare to myself right now, while I am writing this, "I am in a single-minded focus and I am meditating. Instead of thinking about joining the cosmic conversation, which I think is a complex accomplishment, I just need to practice a still mind, with one thought, not 10, and this is my foundation."

When we approach a difficult task with patience, visualizing the smaller tasks first, putting the big picture aside for a moment, the task becomes more approachable. How did I write a book this dense? I started with the title. I opened the document and started writing page one. I made a commitment to write only one page per day. If I missed a few days, I made up for it when I resumed writing. I maintained the simple task of writing one page per day. Then one day I looked at my book draft and I had written hundreds of pages. The momentum was there.

At that point I was inspired to organize all the topics, and I did so. The next task was to find an editor. The task after that was to find a person who could lay out the book for submission to the printer. I worked on the book by taking on these and other small steps and putting aside any anxiety regarding completion of the finished product.

I made the small steps important. I trusted in this process. Absorb and understand this, and work at improving your life in the same way. Avoid the painful attachment of not being at the "finish line." Be at the starting gate. Then be in your next step. Be content to be working on something. Be in the process. This may take some time to absorb and incorporate. The first step was to read this. The next step may be to think about it. The step after that will be reading it again. Little by little, complete your steps and don't worry if you don't get as far along as you'd like as fast as you'd like. You're going to accomplish your goal, and don't worry if it takes a good while to do so.

5. Maintaining Healthy Dietary Patterns Is a Big Step Towards Self-Mastery

There are a number of concepts that anyone wanting to achieve long-term weight loss and a healthy lifestyle must understand. Some of those concepts may seem esoteric or metaphysical in nature, but understanding them is crucial. A number of positive behavioral changes will be crucial as well. These changes include meditation, writing assignments, dietary improvements, exercise, and prayer, to name a few.

The first concept to consider is that we actually have a relationship with food and that that relationship is likely dysfunctional. We need to mend and improve our relationship with this activity that provides us with energy and ultimately with life. In the process of doing so, we need to understand what we are doing that is out of alignment with our nature. We also need to understand what things have gone wrong with respect to what humans now consider food, how we treat animals for our food, and how food is manufactured, marketed, and distributed throughout the world. This awareness is crucial to being able to complete and sustain a comprehensive recovery.

This understanding is essential because humanity's overall concepts around food are absolute madness. Fixing the world is not your problem. However, escaping the proverbial asylum is. It's a problem easy to solve by simply becoming aware of the suffering humanity causes itself and other creatures. Then, stop participating in it. Easier said than done! Humanity's deeply ingrained false assumptions about diet have made us sick as a species and have adversely impacted our world drastically in many, many ways. A couple of examples are outrageous amounts of single-use plastics used to wrap low-nutrient, toxic foods that are adrift in our once pristine oceans and a tremendous number of swollen landfills spanning the globe.

You are now on a journey to break free from the system that we all were indoctrinated into and to develop new ways of thinking. These new ways tie into your overall success with your desire to change your diet and lifestyle patterns. Following is a brief summary of some of the false notions about food that currently prevail on our planet:

1. Food should come from a factory.
2. Animal protein is a solution to the world's hunger problem.
3. Animals were placed here to be enslaved by us and their bodies can be used for whatever purpose we see fit, and no amount of cruelty to them is too great.
4. Protein is a solution for every physical problem we encounter.
5. Fruit is bad for us and not an essential part of our daily food intake.
6. Vegetables are a side dish.
7. Processed food is so convenient that even though it's a scourge on mankind and on the planet, its manufacture and use is acceptable.
8. Drugs and surgery are there for us to continue unhealthy lifestyle patterns because they can fix us right up.
9. Food is a device we can use to repress feelings such as anxiety.

So much has gone wrong that it's hard to decide where to begin in describing the problems. These problems are interconnected. Governmental regulating bodies allow food corporations to package and label toxic food. Supermarkets and other stores sell such food without consciousness of the damage their industry causes. People, even those who are well-meaning, raise their children by feeding them things that produce lifelong cravings for addictive and destructive foods. Other problems include issues pertaining to the human psyche, the relationship that we in the modern world have with our planet, and the unique obstacles that each individual encounters while on a path towards self-improvement.

You have to ask yourself: What is the level of my individual desire for self-mastery? It should go beyond just the desire for weight loss. We all should want to reach our higher power. We all should want to be the best that we can be.

To succeed in doing so, we must learn more about true human nature—that which goes beyond ourselves. Exploring our own human nature enables us to better understand our deficiencies as individuals and as a species. One such deficiency—perhaps the foremost one—is that of our child-rearing practices. If other species reared their offspring in ways similar to the ways that we do, they would become extinct.

It is my strong opinion that everything that becomes broken in the human mind happens during the formative years of our life. I link the damage done to our children to everything terrible that happens to humanity, to its creatures, and to the world.

If we were focused on rearing our children and teaching our peers ways of living that were applicable to our potential for higher consciousness, things in the world would be quite different. We would teach self-worth, self-love, self-esteem, the need for a harmonious relationship with the planet, proper relationships with food, the need for exercise, and the necessity of frequent meditation. These things would be revered as the tools that would enable us to survive and flourish.

We human beings need continuous step-by-step training—from the day we are born until the day we die. We should never stop learning. We should never stop practicing at life.

The most critical time of training is that which takes place during the first 20 years of our lives. This foundational training is crucial—it's the Boot Camp of Life. This training doesn't guarantee that we won't have a variety of struggles, but it should prepare us to deal with those struggles as they arise. I repeat what myriads of others have said: Our training has gotten far away from what is right.

The possibilities of what we could create are limitless, but many things that we create do not serve our best interests. One example: We don't need fast food restaurants that serve nothing but incredibly unhealthy, toxic garbage. Such places are a blight on humanity.

We can certainly revel in the advancements (scientific and otherwise) that we've made. But it is a huge mistake to see everything that looks like progress as actually being progress. We have a tendency to marvel at our technological advancements without considering the short- and long-term consequences of them. If that wasn't the case, then we wouldn't have pharmaceutical medications with negative side effects that far outweighed those medications' benefits. And there are countless other tragic examples of products and technologies that are harmful to us.

6. You're a Pig!

We are not felines, canines, or grassland grazers. Therefore, we cannot sustain eating in the same way that those animals do. Did you know that humans are omnivorous creatures, with a diet more similar to that of pigs than to the diet of any other animal? Humans and pigs consume the widest variety of bioavailable matter, both natural and unnatural.

But we differ from pigs in a certain way: **Unlike humans, pigs will always instinctively make the better food choice when given the option.**

No other animal will make the dietary mistakes that we make! We make lifestyle choices (dietary and otherwise) based on emotions, addictions, and the need to fulfill cravings. Those choices are often not what's best for our biological needs.

We are also misinformed. The food industry and our society support ridiculous ideas about nutrition and medicine.

••

Many medicines prevent us from suffering many of the horrible consequences of our poor eating habits. Therefore, we collectively fail to learn the lessons that those consequences should teach us.

••

Additionally, most people are depleted of their vital energy force because of poor food choices. Vital force, an enhancement to the immune system, is the energy supply that is left over after all of your daily activities, including digestion of food. When you have more energy than is needed to carry out daily activities and are a biologically cleaner organism (which results from making wise lifestyle choices), you acquire this energy reserve. That reserve is helpful to your immune system.

So what is the ideal diet for humans? Should we be eating bananas all day like our ape cousins do? Should we be ravenous meat-eaters like the big cats? Or are we designed to graze like cattle? **None of the above.**

We are actually similar to pigs, bears, and piranhas. We are omnivores. However, we have longer digestive transit times than most other animals. That's why flesh foods are not ideal for us: Flesh foods easily ferment or rot in our digestive system because they stay there too long. Eating anything and everything is possible, but not optimal for longevity.

Indigenous tribes and rural Japanese fishermen are healthier than most other people because they eat smaller portions of food obtained from pristine environments. Their intensely rich spiritual worldviews also play a major role in their success (dietary and otherwise) and long life spans. But we do not live in the same conditions that they do.

We live with pollution, stress, and tainted food supplies. What's worse, nearly everything we eat is processed. In the modern diet, our systems are burdened with processed foods that require enormous force to digest.

That's why we need to assist our natural bodily cleansing and detoxing processes with full fasts, juice fasts, colonics, meditation, writing, talking to others, religious or spiritual practices, and other measures. There are many ways to cleanse and many aspects of our being that continually need cleansing or detoxing. This is called healing, and we do it every moment of every day.

The ultimate way to cleanse as it pertains to diet is to first leave out processed foods. Doing so will allow the mechanisms of the body to take over and do what they were designed to do: Heal!

You can assist in the healing process by doing juice cleanses of durations ranging from six hours to 30 days—whatever you can mentally handle. Also, incorporate more raw foods, smoothies, and pure unadulterated supplements into your everyday diet. (This will be covered in detail in Part Four: The Dietary Change Work.)

Modern science is behind in the area of nutrition, and is sometimes mistaken regarding other health-related matters: Keep in mind the example of scientists and doctors who believed that smoking was not particularly unhealthy back in the 1950s.

It is not the goal of this program to convert people into vegans, vegetarians, flexitarians, etc. You've got to decide where you want your calories and nutrients to come from. Having said that, the problem I have with most nutrition books and diets is that they pander to what they believe the reader will follow and respond to positively, rather than just presenting fact-based scientific data.

One such fact is that no human ever became ill from an iron deficiency, anemia, or a similar malady from abstaining from flesh foods such as red meat, chicken and fish. If a person converts to a plant-based diet and later has deficiencies, 100% of the time it is because they are not getting enough calories from a broad spectrum of produce.

Moreover, just because a person converts to a vegetarian or vegan diet does not mean they discontinued other major dietary mistakes such as eating processed food, which can contribute in an enormous way to various ailments and other health-related problems.

So, while I am not trying to convert people to a plant-based lifestyle, I feel that I do need to defend it because there is so much misinformation being perpetuated about one of the most rational conclusions to draw from evidence-based observations: Plant-based diets are great. Like most things in this world, the devil is in the details. If you execute a plant-based diet poorly, you will have poor results. If you do not get the small details right in any diet, there may not be a wide margin for error for you.

Depending on your overall chemistry, you may get away with murder in your diet. While some suffer greatly when they make the tiniest dietary mistake, others do not. Everyone has a different mindset. Everyone has a different threshold for discomfort. And everyone has deep-rooted beliefs regarding what they're supposed to be eating.

Sometimes those beliefs are rooted in misinformation or incorrect data. One such example is as follows: A doctor may advise a patient to eat more red meat in order to get more iron. That piece of advice was based on information that was incorrectly believed by the medical community at a certain point in time.

There was a time when people believed that red meat was the best source of iron, that cow's milk was the best source of calcium, and that fish oil was the best source of omega vitamins. And people still think that protein is a solution to every physical problem. It's not.

It's crazy to think I lived in an era during which the best scientific minds could not put two and two together and write a comprehensive book on ending food addiction, obesity, food-related illnesses, and food-related suffering of other types. There's simply not enough great knowledge out there yet for the truth seeker to rely on fully.

The goodsugar Diet™ is a precise, focused and detailed approach to eating and living that will positively impact your body chemistry. The main premise of this dietary approach is to eliminate mistakes and rely on plants for most or all of your dietary needs, beginning with getting enough calories. If you follow the concepts in this program you will almost certainly succeed in your weight loss and weight control goals.

The factors beyond this diet's control of your success are your genetic makeup, your overall emotional state of being, and environmental situations that you may be exposed to (e.g., water and air pollution). **Your health will improve immediately for every mistake that you leave out of your diet.** It bears repeating that your limitations for improvement will be equal to the types of mistakes that you leave in your diet and your overall lifestyle, and any problems that stem from environmental and genetic factors.

7. Starting a New Diet Creates Hope

The feeling of hope changes our chemistry in a positive and empowering way. Take a moment to feel hopeful and use that feeling, if you can find it, to catapult yourself in a new direction. Every time you sit to read this book, start with closing your eyes and taking a deep breath in while thinking and feeling the word "hope."

It can be scary to try to overcome an addiction or change a habit that doesn't serve you well. Deciding to embark on a program of radical change may seem overwhelming. This is so not only because it is overwhelming, but also because you know how deeply connected you are to that addiction or well-worn behavior pattern.

There are two types of addictions. One type is physical and the other type is purely psychological. Physical addictions include drugs, alcohol, adrenaline, and even food. Psychological addictions include a wide variety of things, some as simple as obsessively looking at your phone. All psychological addictions have a direct impact on the physical body: They can make us feel elevated, depleted, or both.

I have a life concept that I am asking you to believe in. Believing it will empower you to completely overcome your addiction. The concept is this: No matter what type of addiction you have, you can overcome it if you take the right steps.

In order to fix your problem, you **must** break down the steps that will lead you towards fixing that problem. If you do not know what those steps are, then you can use someone else's step-by-step system. Mine "looks like" what I am about to describe, but yours may be different.

••

The first step is to surrender. You must admit that you have a problem. You must verbalize it (say it out loud), write it down on paper in some detail, and share what you've written with someone you trust. I repeat— You must admit that you have a problem. If you don't acknowledge that you have a problem, you will have no hope of overcoming it.

••

The next step is moving ourselves into a state of quiet and stillness. Some consider such talk to be esoteric hippie mumbo-jumbo, but it isn't. Give it a shot—you have nothing to lose.

Try this:

- ▶ Sit quietly in nature and spend 45 minutes concentrating on your breathing. To some people, the idea of sitting still for 45 minutes seems impossible, so break that down into smaller increments if you need to. Try sitting for three minutes, and then when three minutes becomes easy, try to sit for five, and so on. Even if you only sit quietly for three minutes you will get a benefit.

- ▶ Visualize yourself unhooking yourself from your addiction, habit, or compulsive behavior pattern.

- ▶ See yourself in your thoughts, free from the nightmare of addiction of any kind: See yourself as being truly free. This is the new behavior pattern starting!

The more frequently you can practice sitting still and quiet, even if it's in your closet, the more powerful and positive the impact will be. When I do so, I might be ridiculed by people who say, "Look, there's Marcus sitting in the closet, visualizing himself giving up a habit." But I don't care about public opinion (or private opinion, for that matter). I care about improving myself by systematically discarding my bad habits.

Some consider yoga to be ridiculous. Yoga requires that you do headstands and hold a posture for three minutes to effectuate change. But if you are serious about self-improvement, you must think outside of the box, and if need be try techniques that seem "new agey" and weird.

••

Doing things that seem odd or uncomfortable is preferable to sitting at home suffering and wondering how to make yourself better.

••

When you've become willing to surrender, after you've sat and visualized yourself free from your addiction, the next step is to get out a journal and start writing. Write about how you quit, how you're going to quit, how you may struggle, and/or your connection to the addiction— just write, write, and then write some more. You can use a computer or a pad of paper, whichever you prefer. Writing was and is a big part of my personal recovery and problem-solving actions. (I will cover this more in Part Two: The Primary Work.)

Most of us have addictions buried very deep in our subconscious minds that we don't tap into. One of mine was movement. I needed to be constantly moving in order to feel at peace. I was terrible with stillness unless I was sleeping, and even then I wasn't still. I was also addicted to changes of scenery. I needed my visuals to change frequently: I got bored or frustrated if I saw or encountered the same things every day. My constant movement created unnecessary chaos. I was actually addicted to chaos.

As I got older I learned how to create balance. I learned that I didn't really need for the scenery to change. Instead, I could change the state of my restless mind. I could bring my mind to wherever I wanted it to be. I learned that I could become happy while looking at a brick wall every day if I had no other choice.

Coming to such a state of mind is not easy. But I am at the point now where I can do things that I need to do, such as shop and go to work, and enjoy the changes of scenery rather than be addicted to them. My practices of meditation helped me a great deal with that particular struggle. And I want to stress that meditation will help you a lot in your journey to overcome whatever addictions or obsessions you may be struggling with too.

It is my fervent desire that some of the things that I will suggest in this book—in addition to the crucial entities of admission, surrender, and calming of the mind—will help you attain great physical and mental health, and much hope, happiness, and inner peace.

The various steps that you will need to take will be described in the remainder of this book. They will help you to control your weight and discontinue your unhealthy eating patterns. The steps need not be followed in a precise sequence. But I very strongly recommend that you do each and every one of them and review them all frequently.

As meditation is particularly important, I'd like to conclude this short section by describing a simple meditation exercise appropriate for beginners:

Sit quietly for five minutes, three days per week. Visualize yourself in a better place. Visualize yourself being free from whatever unpleasantness your obsession or addiction may have brought into your life. Visualize any unpleasantness in your life as being something that will change. Sit or lay down and do quick breathing exercises with long inhalations, focusing on the word hope and its core Google Dictionary definition: Hope is "*a feeling of expectation and desire for a certain thing to happen.*"

As stated on *hopegrows.net*, a website I thought was pretty good at defining this, "**To have hope is to want an outcome that makes your life better in some way.** *It not only can help make a tough present situation more bearable but also can eventually improve our lives because envisioning a better future motivates you to take the steps to make it happen.*"

8. Get Excited About Starting Your Journey

As I stated earlier, your journey to accomplish your goals has already begun. You've come to the point of realizing that issues in your life need attention so that you can live a healthier life moving forward.

This indicates emotional and psychological maturity on your part. You're moving past the roadblocks that you encountered in childhood, when admitting mistakes constituted blows to your ego that you couldn't handle. You may have blamed other children and adults for your problems—for the ways that you were making your own life more difficult all by yourself.

During childhood, it's our parents' responsibility to provide a loving, safe environment and to instill emotional maturity. If they didn't do so, we often developed personality problems evidenced by our not taking responsibility for mistakes of our own making. When we're not able to recognize our own mistakes, we stay stuck in our own suffering.

Writing is a powerful tool for helping you achieve the positive change that you seek and is crucial to effect positive change—I cannot emphasize this enough. It's been absolutely invaluable to me for 35 years, and I've seen it work wonders for countless others as well.

I'd like to give a few details about how you can begin this process. The first step is to write down all of the problems that you've had in your life up until this moment. Write down whether or not they have been solved. For any problems that still exist, write down what you think you might be doing that keeps you from solving those problems.

After you've written down your various problems, you can study what you've written and move closer to solving those problems, one by one. As an example, suppose you're having a problem with your ex-wife. You can look at your entry and consider what you are doing to make the situation worse, asking yourself what your part is in the conflict. Recognizing a problem and considering how you may be exacerbating it will provide a fuller understanding and move you closer to a solution.

You may wonder what this has to do with shedding a few pounds—why an academic exercise could help with weight loss or weight control. The reason is that all of our addictions are directly connected to our anxieties. Our anxieties are in turn connected to our fears that we had as children. Those fears are amplified in the re-creation of our childhood during our grown-up life.

In order for us to move forward, we have to get to the place where we are truly emotionally healed. If you follow the steps, work on meditation, and improve your diet, there's a 300% chance you're going to feel at least 60-100% better than you did before.

Because you are reading this, right here and right now, it means that your journey to weight control and a healthy lifestyle has begun. Be happy, excited, and encouraged about this.

A roadblock or trap for some is that their weight control problems seem overwhelming. Weight problems won't disappear overnight, and this discourages such people. This is the case because they lack patience. They need to learn to focus on the short-term goals of taking daily steps toward weight control and healthier living. One of the golden rules of mastering addictions and problem behaviors is the necessity of learning how to live day by day. This principle is a cornerstone of programs such as Alcoholics Anonymous, and this book will dive further into strategies on how to live that way.

We generally take time for granted. But we should wake up every single day and tell ourselves that today is the only day in our lives. So, I advise you to repeat the following phrase (or words to the effect of the phrase) to yourself over and over again: "Today is my only day. I will work to make my day exactly as I want it to be. I'm doing that so that I can appreciate today and be in it. I want my day to go exactly as I dream it. This is within my control."

You made it this far in the book. Please continue. There's a lot of good stuff coming, and it will help you tremendously.

As we endeavor to free ourselves from our obsessions with food or weight problems, we have to set our intentions every day to gently win over our lower impulses. We have to be forgiving of ourselves because we struggle sometimes.

You can do this food thing right. You can be victorious if you believe in yourself, starting today, starting right now.

Say to yourself over and over and over: "I believe I can do this. I can master this area of my life. I want to be happy. I want to feel and be healthy. I want to feel joy (or more joy). I want to share joy. I want to help others."

9. This Book Will Help You—I Guarantee It

The primary purpose of this writing is to help you fight your battle against unhealthy eating patterns. The book deals more with mental and emotional processes than it does with things such as calorie counts and specific foods. The diet that you will eventually embrace will be one that is tailored to your own needs, practices, and disciplines. And it's likely to be one that includes a great deal of vegetables, fruits, nuts, sprouts, and seeds, and little or no animal protein.

You might expect any book on nutrition to have an entire section that explains how cells cluster together and form the tissues of your body and how the tissues cluster together to form organs. Many books about nutrition go into very deep detail about molecular science.

This is not that kind of book, one reason being that I'm not an expert on those subjects. My friend Dr. Jeffrey Mechanick is an expert; he wrote two books on molecular nutrition for the medical community. I've gone to him often over the years to get information. He is second to none in terms of being an authority in chemistry pertaining to nutrition. He states unequivocally that the most important thing that a person can do for their health is to study their own dietary patterns and make changes to them in order to correct mistakes.

The goodsugar Diet™ is more about teaching us what not to eat and not overemphasizing the specifics of what to eat on a moment-by-moment basis, because that can oftentimes get very confusing. I have found that people become enlightened when they concentrate on what they should be leaving out of their diet, because then the choices of what to eat become easier.

So, in this model, you are reducing your choices, and by doing so making it harder for you to make dietary mistakes. The first reaction most people have when they hear that they have to eliminate foods from their diet is that they start to hold on a bit tighter, resisting changing their behavior. They start to negotiate with themselves; they want to moderate, not eliminate.

If we believe that we can moderate the extremely highly addictive and toxic foods in our diet, we will not succeed. We must come to terms with the fact that certain food groups cannot be moderated—they need to be eliminated completely. A little poison is still poison.

For too long, the "diet world" has been focused on things such as calorie consumption and amounts of processed sugar in particular products. This guide offers an entirely different model. It encourages you to determine how much nutritional value is in the products you are consuming, calorie for calorie. Look for the good, not less of the bad.

This book's intent is also to make you aware of the early days of eating, referring to smart human beings who lived close to the land and honored all aspects of its giving. These people weren't tearing things out of packages, and they weren't eating foods laden with harmful chemicals.

Throughout history, mankind's circumstances have differed from continent to continent and from climate to climate. In much colder climates, people had to rely on animal protein because they didn't have UPS and Federal Express to ship superfood powders from Colombia to New York. They didn't have refrigerated trucks to drive cucumbers from Mexico to Washington, DC. So people ate in accordance with the seasons and what the soil would bear. If the soil would bear nothing, then people lacking technologies capable of changing that would be driven to animal protein by necessity.

People ate what the forests or the jungles would put into their paths. Sometimes that would be the flesh of an animal or an insect. Those same people were always breathing clean air and drinking pure water, both free from chemical compounds that would harm their bodies. They were extremely active as individuals, they collectively had a great sense of daily purpose, and they had rich spiritual and metaphysical world views. These things generally resulted in positive attitudes and respect for the present moments being experienced by these early ancestors of ours.

It's very unfortunate that most of us in the modern world have lost those good things, to varying degrees. They are not lost forever—they're just lost for the moment. We have only lost touch with these things temporarily.

It's vitally important for anyone embarking on a journey to healthier dietary practices, including weight loss, to first understand some fundamental concepts about unhealthy eating patterns. Concepts such as the psychological, sociological, spiritual, and intellectual reasons behind unhealthy eating patterns, plus some specific scientific principles. Such information will be the primary focus of this book.

10. What Kind of Eater Are You?

This question requires reflection and contemplation on your part. As I will explain in the next few chapters, I think this is a moment for you to begin a journal where you can write about how you relate to your food—how you've always related to food. This is the beginning of self-realization.

There are two types of eaters that I have observed. The first type is madly, madly in love with the process of eating: They love to excite their taste buds, they love to sit at the dinner table, they love a good conversation, they love being full, and they love what their eyes see when they look at food. They may need for most of their meals to feel like an event and to be something incredibly soothing.

This first type of eater might have very deep emotional connections to the process of eating. They might have been really connected to their families at meals during holidays. Most of their joyous memories encompassed the food that was present in those interactions. They must have really embraced and enjoyed the love of their family and being surrounded by food in all directions.

Many of us enjoyed such positive connections with food and family. But at the same time, there may have been a lot of drama and dysfunctional dynamics unraveling during these mealtimes and gatherings. For many of us, there was just too much food: Food on every table, food in every closet, and bags and plates of junk food everywhere you looked.

Some of us grew up in homes where during holidays (sometimes as often as once a week) members of the family would just sit down and gluttonize. This is what I experienced growing up, and I had to unlearn that as a pattern in my own life.

The second type of eater does not see food as anything particularly special. They eat when they get hungry, perhaps they overeat, or perhaps they eat when they're in a rush or when they're anxious. They may not have such a deep connection with the joy of food, but they need the chemical reaction of eating, whatever it may be. This type of eater may be too divorced from the Zen and joy of eating: This too could be a problem.

When you go through the exercise of determining the type of eater that you are, it will make it easier to understand what you feel you're missing and what you will need later during the processes of unlearning and relearning. I think that there's a healthy balance that we can write about and discuss with our closest confidantes. The balance comes from the place between eating just for pleasure and eating just for survival purposes.

....

When you are attempting to fix any problem that you have in your life, it's usually a slow process with many setbacks along the way. However, if you have had those setbacks already, and are still struggling, you may be ready to try the suggestions in this book. They can liberate you from an eating problem, but getting the energy and courage to start doing them is your challenge. But you can do it!

....

There's nothing wrong with taking some comfort in food. Food is a blessing. It feels great, it keeps us alive, and we should celebrate it. But we have to keep everything in our lives in perspective and in balance. We can't allow the comfort of food to completely overwhelm us. We can't get to the point where we cannot find comfort unless we are in the rapture and passion of food and eating. We can't allow ourselves to be overtaken by cravings.

We will talk later in the book about the sources of eating problems. These include difficulties that we experienced in our childhoods, trapped emotions, and deep-seated character problems.

11. What Is Self-Improvement?

The discipline of taking care of the tedious tasks of life can be applied to all aspects of life—we are seeking presence of mind during all actions that we take. We want to be truly where we are at any given moment. This is the key to experiencing happiness.

I define self-improvement as taking on the difficult tasks that we need to manage by ourselves, and for ourselves, every day of our lives—until they become habits. Once these positive actions become habits, then you'll do them without even needing to think about them anymore. Self-improvement starts with the ability to see our shortcomings, and having the positivity and strength to do the work that it takes to improve them. Self-help does not mean we need to do everything alone. We still need people. We need our support, whether it's from books and therapists, friends, relatives, or other sources. Self-help is helping ourselves to begin to change for the better.

We need to do the first bits of work. We need to buy the book that will help us; we need to lift it up, open it, and read it. We need to admit that we have a problem with diet, weight control, or food addiction. Then we need to get into the solution and make it become a reality—no one can do that for us. Self-help also entails us finding the support groups and the appropriate support people, calling on and interacting with God (if we have such belief), and finding the right resources and companions.

It's also important to note that self-improvement is a measurement of personal success. Success is a steady journey that has brought us from where we were to where we now find ourselves.

Personal success has nothing to do with how much money you've acquired, how many promotions you've received, and the like. Personal success is measured by how well we can improve ourselves and address our own specific challenges, all the way to the very end of our lives!

Cleaning up behavior patterns that pertain to healthy lifestyle choices and diet is extremely difficult. When you finally do it and feel safe with it, it will be a major accomplishment. It will be as big as anything that you have ever done in your entire life.

Achieving the relationship with food that we would like would have been easier if we came from a lineage of people who understood the land, its fertility, and how to cultivate healthy foods. A lineage who didn't have the types of traumas and anxieties that we have in our societies today. These traumas and anxieties are so prevalent in our societies today that we are often desensitized to their presence.

Traumas and anxieties make us susceptible to addictions that we use to relieve the discomfort and numb the pain. Most of the problematic events occurred when we were little, when the feelings were so much more intense than they would be today. We now need to address our past problems individually, one by one, and then collectively as a society.

There are a number of requirements for successful self-improvement, and two in particular are extremely important: Recognizing that that life improvement is needed and having a strong desire to make it happen. Self-help requires that an individual has a lot of drive. After beginning the process, determination to stay with the process is necessary. This requires long-term focus.

Practices such as meditation, writing, therapy, prayer, and other things help a person keep focused for the long term. Self-help requires discipline, courage, patience, and fervent desire. Each new day in the journey, one must be willing to stay on the right path.

No single thing or entity will give you these attributes. You either have them or you have to develop them. If you don't have them to begin with, you can strive to acquire them.

The proper starting point is a degree of self-esteem. Even if you have very little, what you have will help keep you going. If you're struggling to keep yourself going, then you have to first rebuild your self-esteem and then you can continue with discipline and staying on the self-improvement path. Building self-esteem is a complex process that will be somewhat different for each of us. Reading books such as this one will help.

Some people attempt to boost their self-esteem by acquiring possessions such as beach houses and hot sports cars, which usually benefit them only temporarily. A true solid foundation of self-respect and dignity should be based on two things: That we exist, and that we want to be happy. If you're missing these things, then you need to dive deeper psychologically and emotionally to find out where they went.

Think long and hard about the word discipline. It has nothing to do with punishment in this case. In the context of self-help, it has to do with our practicing positive repetitive behavior regardless of how we feel.

Generally speaking, if we have addictions it means that there are areas of our lives that were missing discipline. So we then try to train our minds to become disciplined. This is a big step, but as is the case with many things, the easiest way to take on big steps is to try to break them down into smaller and smaller ones. Every day we should take at least one step toward self-improvement.

A step forward, no matter how tiny, is still progress. I will say it again and again: A big step in your long-term self-help program is learning how to break big steps into smaller ones. This is especially important when you reach an impasse: Tell yourself that you will move forward little by little and improve yourself as a person as you do.

The repair of our lives begins with our thoughts. The right thoughts lead to our speaking the right words. Then, we take the right actions. Such actions include the development of skills to improve thinking—practices such as mindful meditation. This appropriate action also includes finding and dealing with old emotions that are hidden within us yet still plague us. Doing so is something that is likely to take a considerable amount of time.

12. We Must Be Honest With Ourselves

We must see ourselves honestly. We can't fix what is broken inside of us unless we do that.

Many of us, perhaps most of us, had difficult childhoods. It is crucial to identify the most traumatic experiences of our childhoods and then consider how our responses to those experiences affect our adult behavior. But doing so isn't easy. We often just can't see the deeper meaning behind certain behaviors that we have and how those behaviors are affecting our world.

In a very real sense, we're still little children trying to enter into the world of adult reality. And we get stuck in the process—we have a hard time transitioning from one phase of life to another. This is the case because we experienced so much crisis in these phases during which emotional growth was arrested.

But, thankfully, there is a solution. Start by writing the word "self-awareness" in your journal. What does self-awareness mean? Self-awareness begins with the ability to quiet the mind and take a journey with your words. You must focus intently to figure out who you are and what you are doing.

You must then ask yourself many questions. Some of them are as follows: What are your philosophies? What are your beliefs? What do you think you know? What judgments do you make that hold you back from moving forward? Are you brave, or do you think that you're a coward? Do you love deeply, or are you so stuck that you can't feel love? Are you a person who feels horny a lot, or never, or an average amount? Do you feel lonely most of the time, or do you feel connected to people? What are all the good characteristics that you can describe about yourself without being egocentric? What do you think the world needs most from you? These and other things are very important self-reflections.

I would like to ask you to write down the following words in your biographical journal, because the path to happiness is actually as simple as reading the words and repeating them over and over:

- ▶ **Your life is wonderful.**
- ▶ **Everything that you've encountered is a miracle.**
- ▶ **Every second to come is a blessing.**

Some people have never had or rarely have had kind words spoken to them. Let these kind words plant seeds in your mind and let those seeds grow. Hearing these words and experiencing their positive effects grows with time within us.

If we want to change we must do a number of things daily, such as becoming aware of our self-destructive behavior and strongly resolving to discontinue it. Think about overcoming it, talk about overcoming it, and do good things each and every day that will make the process of overcoming it a reality. These are the behaviors that are going to set you free. They will help you lose weight, and they will help you to want to eat healthier.

Changing your negative, problematic thinking patterns may not happen overnight. But if you are fiercely committed to that process of change, it can begin happening soon. You can find a degree of relief as soon as right now.

13. This Is a Challenging, Worthwhile Journey You Will Succeed At

Before you continue on with this book, I want to acknowledge how difficult dietary change is. It doesn't make a difference how old we are, how overweight we might be, or what medical problems we may have, weight control can be difficult.

I know that if you're reading this book you want nothing more than to reach your goal of controlling your weight. To me, weight loss is secondary to mental and physical health. But for most people it is the primary driver, and I know that nothing I say will change that. So you may pursue the steps I am describing with weight loss as your primary driver if you wish to do so.

If that's the case, though, at least put it in your mind that your secondary driver is that you want to be physically healthy. The third driver should be that you want to master yourself—your emotions, your consciousness, and your overall mental health. And in that self-mastery you want to feel good in your body and feel good about your time here on earth.

••

Train yourself from the very beginning to not have your measure of success be completely based on whether or not you lose weight.

••

14. Distraction and Lack of Good Habits

Throughout my life I found myself working hard at "self-helpy" types of things. Today it's easy for me to see that the two things that trip me up the most are: (1) distraction; and (2) a lack of routine in the areas in which I need positive change.

I get distracted by all kinds of things, some of which lead me astray. In addition to the lack of focus to stay on a particular path, I did not make the necessary things into routines and habits. The lack of focus combined with the lack of ingrained habits means I am prone to falling away— even from small things such as being kind and thoughtful. Thankfully, a great teacher taught me that meditation would build my focus, keep me calm, and help me to not be negatively affected by various troubles.

Repetition will fix my need for building habits and crushing laziness. Laziness is always linked to fear. Half of everything we think may be naturally linked to fear, and the other half to a true sense of oneness. We get so distracted from that oneness, and the sense of safety that it brings, that the only place to move into is fear. This is normal. But the events of our formative years will determine if the 50/50 ratio becomes skewed more toward fear or more toward oneness.

15. Practice, Not Perfection

In order to get to the next level with solving our problems, we've got to take action of some kind. We can't wait until we figure out all of our childhood problems, free all of our trapped emotions, and only then take action. It's unrealistic to think that our lives begin only when we are perfect. We will never be perfect in this life. Our lives are practices. We can achieve progress during our lives, but not perfection.

PART TWO
THE PRIMARY WORK

16. Create a Journal and Always Write in It

The most profound action we can take each day to participate in our happiness is writing. It is not important that you become a wordsmith, a poet, or a cherished novelist. Writing is an action that takes thoughts, goals, problems, solutions, ideas, pathways, and other entities from being disorganized to becoming organized. It takes these entities from being imaginary to being real, and from the internal world to the external world for our further examination and contemplation.

Talking with and listening to others is the most valuable way of getting in touch with feelings and learning how to deal with them. But what does a person do if they're alone? What does a person do if they shut down and they don't know what they feel? What should a person do if they don't have anyone to talk to?

They should write.

And you should write, whoever you are, whatever your situation is, and whether or not you have people who you can talk with. You can call the bulk of what you write a journal or you can call it whatever you like. Writing is a very powerful action. Anything that you write is actually you taking a step and taking an action in order to improve your situation.

Writing is one of the most essential tools for recovering your emotions and letting them move through you. You take vague memories and abstractions that are in your head and put them on a piece of paper or on the screen of your laptop. This quickly crystalizes things.

Then you can begin digging into your deepest feelings and determine their earliest connections. The more you write about a situation, the more you're likely to find a feeling attached to it. Even if you can't find a feeling attached to it, you can write about how you cannot feel.

When I cannot feel an emotion attached to a memory I journaled about, I look at the entry days later. When I read it back to myself out loud, I might say, "I think I am supposed to be saddened by this thing I just wrote about, but I don't feel anything." Then I write about why I think I can't feel certain emotions. I create a dialogue with myself to trace an emotional issue or problem to its root cause.

This is the power of journaling—enabling you to determine your feelings, focus on them, and take steps to heal. That healing then makes you able to live a happier, healthier, and more productive life.

When I started writing, I could not believe how much difficult content I was able to find that had been lost somewhere in my mind. Only writing could pry open my worst thoughts and gently preserve my best thoughts. I write my strategies and plans on how I will solve a problem in detail. I give myself instructions in my writing.

You can use your writing the same way that I do or go about it somewhat differently if you prefer. Write about feelings experienced during the day. Write an instruction booklet on how to make friends. Write about a resentment you have, write about the mysteries of life. The process of writing itself is cathartic. In other words, the writing provides mental and emotional relief through the free expression of strong emotions and deep thoughts.

In 12-step recovery, one of the suggestions is to write about your life and then read what you've written to someone else. It's a very powerful step, especially if you continue to do it throughout your life.

Journaling does not have to consist of 1,000-page-long essays. Perhaps you're sitting by your computer working, and suddenly a feeling of anxiety comes up. You can just write the word "anxiety" down.

Two entries are crucial, though. The first is your written "admission" statement—this is described in the "Smash Denial: Admit That You Have a Problem" section of this book.

From that point, write a plan on how you will stay away from the addiction and improve the quality of your life. In doing so, you will be writing out your future mission statement. The things that you write will be the things that you look to, meditate on, and actively do when troubles begin to overwhelm your mind. At that point, you will be moving from admission to an understanding of the problem and of taking concrete action steps to overcome it.

Journaling could also be part of the process of writing your entire life story down and then sharing it with your best friend or therapist. If you do write out your entire life story and later find that it's missing major pieces, it will be essential for you to fill in the blanks. It will be difficult to reconstruct the information from memory at a later date if you don't write it down.

Some readers may find that the term journaling or the idea of writing does not sit well with them. I experience that reaction from people who meet with me in person to ask for help. Essentially, they appreciate the talking aspect of a self-help program but are not as committed to doing hard work as they need to be.

Journaling is pertinent to our relationship with food and to weight loss. It circles back to the need for a lifelong commitment to staying with our recovery work and not letting it slip away. The risk of relapse is very high for people such as us.

Our addictions persist because the underlying anxieties and feelings behind them do not dissipate on their own. They need to be worked on daily. Seven days a week. No holidays. Our addictions and difficult emotions do not take breaks. They persist in our lives forever until we deal with them and heal. We need tools to help us do that.

Writing is a crucial tool in this process. It's absolutely necessary, and it's the baseline of recovery. There's a lot more work of other types to do, but writing about everything that we think of is a starting point. It is the liberating action that starts the chain of recovery in motion.

There are three things that will keep us from writing: (1) laziness; (2) fear; and (3) disbelief that the writing will have any benefit. Put those three things aside—they are of no value to you.

Writing is also a valuable distraction for us when we have times when we feel anxious and on the verge of acting out in a negative way—such as addictive eating to stuff our feelings. Instead of going to the fridge right away when you're upset, try writing about your feelings first. This may sound overly simplistic, but it works!

Writing is a way for us to memorialize our healing process. You should write out your current plan of action when you begin your recovery. At a later date when you're farther along in your recovery, compare it to the way you think at that point in time.

If we are complacent for just one day in being mindful of our addictive potential, we are then in peril of being complacent for a second day in a row. In the blink of an eye, 10 days went by during which we did nothing to support our mental health. Thirty days pass, and we are then in a pattern of decline. We are a train slowly heading towards a fractured track somewhere in the distance. If we hit that piece of damaged track, we will likely be derailed and then relapse.

As I mentioned earlier, I never relapsed with drugs or alcohol. I got sober at age 15 and I stayed sober. However, through the years I went through long periods of inaction and I made colossal mistakes. I suffered in many ways. Had I been in therapy, been in a good support group, been journaling, been reading books on recovery, working mediation practices, and taking other steps, I'm certain that I wouldn't have made the bad decisions that led me down some very difficult paths. Not journaling was one of my biggest mistakes.

17. Who Else Journaled Throughout History? You're Not a Dweeb for Writing

Be aware that all of the great thinkers of the last 100,000 years of human history were epic "journalers." They were prolific writers that wrote about everything.

I suggest that when you write, you imagine yourself to be an important person writing to future readers—not just to yourself. See yourself as someone who is creating the world's most captivating movie script in intimate detail.

Socrates, Plato, Einstein, Dubois, Cornel West, Thomas Shelby, Hypatia, Ayn Rand, Buddha, Moses, Cudworth, Aristotle, Descartes, Antebi (just kidding), Nietzsche, Alan Watts, Confucius, Gandhi, Krishnamurti, Vandana Shiva, Swami Prabhupada, countless native American and indigenous philosophers, and many others journaled. These and an infinite number of other great thinkers used writing to document their experiences and their practicing of their philosophies.

When we write about our lives we are validating the dramas and realities of our experiences. This has a profound impact on our self-help personal therapy. Such writing is one of two powerful tools in self-help. The first is writing, the second is talking.

Many of the great philosophers and great historical figures, both male and female, wrote about their lives and ideas. **Write!**

18. Important Writing Assignments

Write out the steps that you think that you need to take to get yourself better. Keep that writing close to your bedside and keep reading it. It's often just a question of getting focused and being able to get yourself back on your adventure wagon. Take all of the actions that I ask of you in this book. If you're overwhelmed by the amount of necessary actions, then you have to further break down the steps that you need to take.

I use such a process when I'm writing something for my work. First, I write a general outline of the steps I need to take to accomplish something in the business. For example, I may need to find a bottling consultant. If I have no idea how to find a bottling consultant, then I write down the step before that. In this case, it would be to call up 10 people who might know a bottling consultant and ask them if they have any contacts. If I don't solve my work-related problems in this way, I will never get the solutions I need and subsequently will never progress and move forward in my business.

Applying this process to a self-help program might look something like this: You write down "Step one: Lose weight." That step is likely not detailed enough.

You probably have to put a number of steps before it. A more realistic first step might be, "Step one: Read that guy's book on weight loss."

Another assignment is as follows. Write the following phrase down in the morning: "It doesn't matter if I'm skinny or overweight—what matters is that I have my addiction under control." Then, say it to yourself several times.

Weight loss and many other very significant benefits will follow over time.

19. The Power of the Task List

You should begin every day with a written list of the things that you need to accomplish.

I suggest that you first pray or meditate briefly, do some breathing exercises, wash your hands and face or shower, drink some water, and then write out the things that you want to accomplish today. This should be your morning ritual.

It's best to start a new list fresh every day. This is because every day that you wake up, you are a new person. You need not be chained to your old ways.

You may add things not yet done from previous days, but your current day's list must be based on your emotions and your physical condition today. Doing this is an integral part of living in the present moment.

•••

Every day's list must include the tasks that you will hold yourself accountable to later. You are accountable to yourself, your happiness, and your goals.

•••

I need to emphasize that the most meaningful changes in my own healing process came for me when I embraced writing and thought of my daily task lists as crucial (rather than just as a pastime).

Certain messages should be associated with your tasks. These messages should encompass being kind to yourself in your writing and kind to who you see when you look in the mirror. Be kind to all others at all times, even those you do not like—even people who are not in your life but in your mind. Say nice things to them or they might contribute to ruining your day, even if they are not present with you.

Examples of things typically on my daily task lists include the following: Listen better when someone is speaking so that I might understand them better. Do not react first, but process first. Breathe and take time to gain my poise before reacting. Ask myself, is my reaction going to ruin my day or cause me calm? Ask myself, will I feel anxious or will I feel okay?

20. The Importance of Saying the Right Words and Taking the Right Actions

We must slowly gain cognizance about what we say in the world. Things that we say become either spells that keep us locked in suffering or magic that frees us. So we have to practice only saying positive words.

Does this take practice? You'd better believe it does! But no matter what happens, you must try to find the positive to get through it. It may not be that a situation is positive. But there are still positive things and positive energies around you.

Having said that, you have to let yourself go through your feelings, especially very negative ones, in order to heal. You have to experience sadness, cry, and overcome that repressed sadness.

But an even more crucial thing is our own monitoring of our behavior. We must make sure that we are saying and doing positive things in the world each and every day.

I have noted that there are three kinds of people in the world. There are people who are saying and doing positive things continually, no matter what is happening. They can feel vibrations of positivity and truth. This type of person understands that everything is passing. Such a person takes control over their time on earth and is always ready to move forward.

The next kind of person is one who is struggling but senses that good and truth are real things that can be achieved. Such people desire to only do good and they want to feel happy. They want to do kind things. They want to create laughter. They want to see and feel the beauty in nature. And they certainly don't want to carry anger around.

Such people may have too many attachments to the wrong things. They may have been conditioned in inappropriate ways, or they may be damaged by difficult childhood experiences. Such trauma isn't often mentioned in ancient philosophies. Since that's the case, adults who had rough childhoods feel disconnected from those extremely valuable teachings from earlier eras.

The third type of person that I know of is one who knows that there is such a thing as right and wrong yet chooses not to do things that are right. Such people prefer bad behavior. They take pleasure in hurting people, hurting things, and hurting themselves. These brothers and sisters suffer. They often suffer to a degree that even competent psychiatric and medical professionals can't help them. But they need your forgiveness, just as you need your own forgiveness for your own shortcomings and transgressions.

21. Celebrate the Beginning of This New Journey

Your life is a celebration, even when there are problems in it. Please take a moment to read that sentence again and feel it in the very core of your being.

The fact that you are looking at these pages, reading a book to improve your life, is extraordinary. Even if you don't find some of the content to be as helpful as you might like, your presence here and now attempting to engage yourself in lifestyle improvement is truly a monumental moment in your life.

Please take a moment and be happy. Even if you allow your misery to sit there waiting around the corner, try to be happy just for a moment. Say to yourself, "I am happy that I am at the beginning of my health and wellness journey."

I believe that you have been on a health and wellness journey since the moment that you were born. Think about how hard you have struggled for your entire life to keep it all together. Take a moment to think about all the times in life that you didn't struggle and things just came together anyway. Try to summon the feeling of gratitude for those times. Gratitude actually has an enormously positive effect on your body chemistry.

I have a fantasy of sorts. It involves my having an infomercial on late night TV. I would present myself as if I was selling superfoods, but what I would really do is sell people things such as gratitude, compassion, fortitude, integrity, honesty, positive attitudes, and happiness. I would elaborate on how those feelings have the same impact for them that drinking celery juice would. I would explain to people how becoming overrun by our negative attitudes is as bad for us as drinking Red Bull and eating

Hostess Twinkies. I would charge lots of money for these states of mind, because people value what they pay for. These things are worth all of the money in the world.

I do understand that we sometimes reach low points with our problems, so much so that we can't seem to take any action. Conscious contact with your higher power will help lift you up from such moments. I firmly believe that, no matter how deep into your problem you may be. You have the capacity to do the writing assignments and continue reading this book. You can break your self-improvement steps into smaller steps that are easier for you to take. If you do so, you will accomplish your goals.

I recommend that you keep this book very close to you at all times. Even if all you can manage to do is read one page a day, start with that. But keep it close and keep coming back to it. Right now, this book represents your willingness to try to tackle your problems, whatever those problems may be.

I think that whenever a person has resolved to embrace self-improvement of any kind, he or she has begun a new and exciting journey. And that journey should not just be a "head trip" filled with lots of deep thinking. The journey should also be a **time of action**, right from the very start.

If you have taken the decisive step of resolving to address your weight control issues, I ask that you take the following action, beginning right now—even before you begin reading the rest of this book:

• •

Draw up a task list of actions that you will take today to improve your life. Make it one item, or make it 50.

• •

Do the same thing at the beginning of every day from this day forward. This is an exercise that you must participate in. Take interest in this task list: This task list is a summary of a big part of your life. This daily action is important, but sometimes it's difficult to adhere to it. This is so because we are naturally lazy.

22. Your Dietary Changes Will Help Stop War and Starvation

I believe that the most effective, profound and lasting approach to weight loss is to deepen one's relationship with food and create new lifestyle patterns pertaining to eating and consuming.

I don't believe in parroting any health guru's lifestyle recommendations, or in jumping on a personal trainer's bandwagon regarding efforts to ensure muscle growth and flattening of the tummy. Such things are short-term solutions, and they are completely ineffective for most of us.

Parroting someone else's ideas on diet and consumption leads us to mass confusion and a society of people who do the following things:

- ▶ Struggle with food and food-related health issues,
- ▶ Suffer from a host of self-esteem issues related to struggles with food,
- ▶ Become disconnected from food sources, causing massive global food problems (resulting in animal cruelty and devastation of the planet), and
- ▶ Fight wars over resources, considering the direction the planet is heading because of climate change. In the future, wars could be fought over clean water and nourishing food supplies, the way we fight over oil and other natural resources today.

What does this way of thinking have to do with your reducing the occurrence of cellulite on the back of your thighs? What does this have to do with slimming down the waistline, or maintaining a "six pack" of abdominal muscles?

It has everything to do with those things, because it addresses food, diet, weight loss, and healthy eating from a more holistic approach. We are not just saying things such as "Stop eating potato chips and your problems will subside."

Although things like that are likely to be part of the truth, they won't empower someone in a food addiction to stop something that may be powerfully satisfying to them. It's necessary to replace food addictions with knowledge and emotional healing.

••

Take a moment to make the connection that the entire world will eventually benefit from you reaching success with all the aspects of your life.

••

Your food journey is just one aspect of your development—a beginning aspect. As you continue to improve, then the other aspects of your life (such as relationships, service to others, and a deep concern about the condition of your planet) begin to open up.

So let's embark on this exciting journey with the understanding that focusing on a 360-degree view of food and eating patterns is both a physical and an emotional effort.

23. Comparing Food Addiction to Other Common Addictions

Food addiction has one significant difference from other types of addictions (e.g., alcohol, tobacco, and drugs).

As an example, an individual might be addicted to cocaine. Once that person quits the drug, he or she is done with it. But a person might instead be addicted to something that they cannot completely get out of their lives once they break the addiction. Some of those things might be money, sex, and, of course, food.

A person with a cocaine addiction can break that addiction and never have contact with the substance again. But it's not realistic to expect a person with a sex addiction to never have sex again, or a person addicted to money to never have money again, or a person with a food addiction to never eat food again.

As far as drugs, alcohol, and tobacco are concerned, it's possible to just stop using them completely. Then, after a (hopefully) short period of time, they cease to be ingrained habits. You don't have to negotiate with them and try to control them. You simply abstain 100% from using them and therefore you are recovered. As long as you do not pick these things back up, they are no longer a problem. The problem is at that point transferred back to the internal world of your emotions.

....

But addictions to food, sex, money, and similar essentials are different. We have to reorganize our relationship to them as vital things in our lives that we continue to use (but must not misuse). Such substances are considerably more complicated to deal with. You

have to learn to moderate your usage rather than abstain from them. Regarding food, we have to eat virtually every day, and so every day we have to have a working program to prevent us from being triggered to use food addictively.

• •

Such a program entails that we get to the root of our mental and emotional problems and work hard to overcome them.

24. Expand Your Consciousness— Everyone's Doing It

In my 96,000 page book that I plan to release in 2050, I will explain what consciousness is in its entirety. But for now, simpler definitions must suffice. In the meantime, I'll work hard on my own development.

We can only overcome our tendency to make behavior-related errors by striving to become people that operate at higher levels of consciousness. We need to seek our own happiness in such a way that it doesn't come at the expense of others or at the expense of our planet.

Our environmental errors are prime examples of how our lack of higher consciousness has been problematic for ourselves and others. Our technological advancements in manufacturing have made it so that the creation of massive amounts of garbage harms everyone on the planet.

Broken people were at the forefront of the creation of this problem. Greed and self-interest blinded the eyes of those who might have prevented much misery, had they exercised social responsibility as they manufactured products and conducted business.

If we work towards becoming more aware of the true nature of things, this will likely lead us to less and less suffering. Expanding our understanding of the world and clarifying our true purpose is one of the few great pieces in the puzzle of our happiness. This entire program is centered around the need to expand both our knowledge and our awareness. Put it in your mind that you are a seeker of such awareness and consciousness, and you will attain it quickly.

25. Become Fully Aware of Your Childhood Experiences—Stop Denying

Learning the truth about what happened to us in our childhood is one of life's more painful experiences. We have to uncover difficult events, and doing so brings up painful feelings that we have been avoiding all our lives.

There are consequences to keeping these experiences and repressed emotions trapped inside. The consequences of such repression are staring back at us in our adult behaviors and all of the complex character defenses we created to protect ourselves. Healing is a process of letting these trapped emotions go and then learning new responses.

The work we need to do on ourselves to move forward begins with walking through the dense forests of our past. It's scary for so many reasons, but there is so much hope that comes from braving through the fears of the unknown.

Becoming conscious and awakening yourself is a joyous experience that occurs as you climb higher to your mountaintop. Self-knowledge is a gift—not a curse—and this work leads us to it. Unconscious patterns hold us back from being truly and sustainably happy, and we need to overcome them.

26. Consciousness Expanding Lifestyle Practices

This book covers a number of the most fundamental aspects of healthy living. Something that will speed up the recovery process tremendously is group therapy or one-on-one therapy. Anyone who is trying to eradicate an addictive cycle should find a group or a therapist who specializes in addictive behavior. The therapist should have some background in 12-step recovery and be well-versed in the foundational aspects of the program that I'm espousing.

These foundational aspects include the following entities:

- Emotional discovery.
- Emotional expression.
- Step-by-step behaviors to process emotions and move through them.
- Behavior modification.
- Behavioral accountability to someone.
- Continued education about the nature of self through meditative processes.
- Physical exercise and self-care routines that keep the body healthy and keep the mind interested in actively pursuing longevity.

I emphasise the point of the last bullet. This program espouses the concept that the healed mind pursues longevity—the healed mind is very focused on survival.

27. The Pursuit of Mental Health Is the Pursuit of Consciousness

A key component of survival is good mental health. Mental and physical health must be integrated rather than treated separately. You can't spend seven days a week in analysis and do little or nothing else. Nor can you spend all your time in the gym lifting weights and give no attention to improving your mental health.

We all need step-by-step instructions. If I had the ability to do so, I would write a book containing one page providing details for each day of a lifespan of 100 years. You could pick up that book each day and read a new page to give you that day's plan. But I don't.

Below is a summary of the steps that I suggest throughout this book that I find to be helpful in a program of recovery; they should all be done, but not necessarily in a specific order.

Admit that you have a problem (e.g., food addiction);

Start a journal to: (1) Write an extensive autobiography; (2) Acknowledge admission of your food addiction problem(s) and associated behaviors; (3) Write out every step required to restore you to optimal thinking and happiness, free from the suffering created in your mind, and (4) Write out all of the addictions you have and become ready to stop doing them.

Create the following lists: (1) People you have harmed; (2) People who have harmed you; (3) Things you love; (4) Things you dislike; (5) A wish list; and (6) A list of solutions to your problems.

Create childhood discovery writings: Write about your childhood traumas and discover the shortcomings of your upbringing. Write down what you remember about the worst moments of your childhood. Share these lists and key writings with another person.

Change or become willing to change your diet in the following ways: (1) Eliminate processed foods; (2) Do not eat late at night; (3) Reduce the amount of protein in general, especially animal protein; (4) Consider going 100% plant-based; (5) Do not follow fad diets; (6) Fall in love with the good sugar in fruit and starchy vegetables; (7) Make carbohydrates your primary source of fuel (i.e., the carbohydrates from fruits and vegetables); (8) Drink clean water; (9) Pay attention to how you combine foods together; (10) Eliminate dairy food from cows; and (11) Eliminate alcohol and tobacco.

28. Move Past Traumatic Experiences by Writing About Them

I often ask close friends to determine if they had wonderful or difficult childhoods and then to write down the worst thing that ever happened to them. And it's through that writing exercise that a lot of people discover truly for the first time that their childhood was not how they wanted to remember it. Breaking through such denial is an incredibly powerful step.

By spending a little bit of time every day contemplating childhood and trying to get in touch with associated emotions, you are doing the first part of necessary healing recovery work.

Depending on how deep your traumas go, you may need professional counseling. Coming face to face with your defenses that were put in place as survival mechanisms must be done cautiously.

Go slow with your emotional healing work—do not press yourself. It takes years of practice to be able to go into a full immersion and stay there. Some people can move very quickly through this work because they have good coping mechanisms. They're often able to cry, which is necessary in intense emotional situations. Some people are very good at getting angry for a moment, then feeling their sadness, and then moving right through it. But when some others touch upon their sadness, they have panic attacks because they feel like it will never pass.

As part of my own recovery work I had to talk to siblings, relatives, and my living parents to help me fill in gaps of things I couldn't remember. I had the idea that because I couldn't remember major portions of my childhood that something really bad had happened. So what I had to do first was to look at my adult behavior, because the adult behavior would lead me to a likely causation.

I regret that it took me so long to really dive into the work, because I've known since I was 15 that my childhood wasn't the best. Since the first time I planted my ass in a chair in an AA meeting at 15 1/2 years old, I've understood how to use the tools needed to get control over addictions.

In my late teens I was in therapy. I went to really difficult child abuse and trauma meetings. I read many applicable books. I was really immersed. But because I didn't have the right direction and necessary attention span, or a psychological and spiritual leader, I floundered tremendously.

I stepped out of doing the necessary emotional healing for a number of years. And even though I stayed clean and sober, much of my behavior was the same as what you'd expect from a person who is actively drunk. But I'm not wallowing in regret; I'm just making mention of a significant behavioral mistake so that as I (and hopefully you as well) move forward I won't make the same mistake again.

I do have one giant regret, though. That regret is that though I had valuable tools for emotional healing work at my fingertips early in life, I didn't really know how to use them. As a result, I think I wasted a lot of precious time. So I regret not being persistent and staying involved in the healing work.

But I am deeply involved in that work now at the age of 51. I have a structured system regarding how I write about my feelings and my childhood traumas, I have my support books, and I have a plan of attack. My plan of attack involves everything that's in this book. I do this work on a daily basis. Seven days a week, no days off.

The quality of my parenting and the quality of my relationship with my wife has improved exponentially over the last two years. That is the time that I really began diving deep into the events of my past and conjuring up the feelings that I knew were trapped inside my body. I felt them constantly, even when I wasn't doing the digging. And what they caused me to do was to feel anxious. That anxiety always took me away from being completely happy.

I don't want anxiety and other negative emotions in my life anymore. And I hope that you will come to a similar desire as you read this book. I hope that you will find the paradigm that I've created and the associated exercises to be useful to you.

I wish you luck on your journey. And I'm very confident that you will take some very significant steps forward on that journey if you read this book through in its entirety.

PART THREE
THE PSYCHOLOGY WORK

29. Losing Weight is Not Just for Vanity—It's for Our Peace of Mind

I want to make something very clear as we go deeper into this book. My purpose is to help any person who doesn't like being overweight to find comfort, not judgement.

I have some good news. Specifically, it's that all of your problems have their origins in your variety of ways of thinking. And it will give you a sense of power to know that no matter what you're experiencing, you can be happy in the midst of those circumstances.

In believing that, you may be pushed to a limit. One might ask, what if a person is diagnosed with stage four cancer? It's awful, it's terrible. How could anyone find any good in it? Or what if a person loses their child in an accident? What if a person loses their job or experiences some type of trauma or terror?

It would be denial to label any situation that is painful and uncomfortable as positive in that moment, because it certainly doesn't feel that way. But what people can do throughout their entire lives is to say to themselves in every situation, "Here I am." When you say those three words, it may take you decades to truly understand them, or you might feel their power the moment that you first say them.

This might be one of the hardest things to achieve in life. It's called acceptance. That word can be somewhat cliché and boring in self-help circles: In my early stages in recovery, when people would talk about acceptance and gratitude, the terms were like four-letter words to me. This was so because of all the hypocrisy I could detect in other aspects of the behavior of the people that I was with. In other words, as a teenager I got the wrong impression of what those words really meant and how powerful they could be.

It is possible to get to a place intellectually and emotionally in which acceptance becomes an automatic response to circumstances. But acceptance does not mean being still and suffering or embracing bad things. Acceptance should be something that you feel—an emotional experience similar to feeling sad or happy. When I feel acceptance about something and it has a chance to absorb into my cells, I become empowered and more ready to act from a higher place. At that point I'm no longer ruled by fear or anxiety.

My experience has shown me that being overweight is physically uncomfortable, for some more so than for others. It hurts self-image and self-esteem, and there are many health risks associated with obesity. But I don't feel that I have to convince anyone what the pros and cons of being at an ideal healthy weight are.

One thing that is rarely talked about is the benefit of overcoming addictions and problems in order to come into a state of expanded consciousness. This simply means becoming able to see much deeper into the nature of reality and understand ourselves better. We will relate better to people, we will relate better to the earth, and we will relate better to all the creatures on it.

If we don't get control over addictions, the side effects include becoming physically and emotionally numb and living life as if we are partially asleep. An active addiction is like having bandages wrapped around your ears and your eyes. You can only see what the world looks like out of the small holes between the bandages.

So it is within the context of taking these troubles out of our lives that we think about losing weight. It's not as if I'm a beauty pageant parent trying to make you into the winning contestant, and I don't care if you look great in a bikini or a speedo.

I've seen that if a person hyper-focuses on the object of losing weight as being the primary objective, then they will struggle with weight for much longer than they need to. If they don't surrender that then they will likely struggle with their weight for their entire life.

I have experienced these struggles personally, and have interacted extensively with others who have had or do have the same issues. One of the primary things that I've learned is that long-term, sustained weight loss happens when people are willing to deal with their associated psychological and emotional issues. For that reason, I will focus a great deal on those aspects of health and wellness, although I will not neglect information pertaining to food choices, physical habits, and the like.

I cannot make any promises regarding exactly how much weight you will lose and the length of time it will take to do it. What I can promise you is that if you follow the steps that I have detailed in this book, you will make substantive progress in improving your physical and mental health. And weight loss will follow.

30. The Psychological Program

In the next several sections, I'm going to outline a program that I suggest that a person should do in order to gain control over a weight-related behavior pattern or food addiction.

Every person is an individual, and everyone will respond to things differently. This is especially true of packaged products like books. A prominent name and a graphically stunning cover might attract buyers, but such things can be deceptive. I won't rely on ploys or gimmicks to communicate my information to you. So I will not try to make a complex subject that requires a lot of work and commitment on the reader's part sound extremely easy.

In the beginning of your journey to recovery of any kind, you don't have the balance or the wherewithal to be able to write out a structured program for yourself. It's difficult to do surgery on yourself; it's hard to concentrate while you're bleeding and in pain.

And that's why you've been acting out. You're likely acting out if you've been in this pain for a long time and you feel numb. The pain is going to come to the surface as you begin your journey. Facing up to the pain is one of the things that will be discussed.

I'm now going to explain the steps that I have used. I have found them to be very helpful to me, and others have found them very helpful in dealing with their food addictions as well.

31. Smash Denial: Admit That You Have a Problem

Definition of Denial: Failure to acknowledge an unacceptable truth or emotion or to admit it into consciousness, used as a defense mechanism.

Is denial an emotion, a philosophy, a physical reaction, a lack of knowledge, or a state of being? It's probably all of those things. I don't think there's any other living creature on this planet that has the mechanism of denial: If you consider the things that set us apart from all the other creatures, denial must be close to the top of that list.

Do we have the ability to be honest and truthful about what we're doing at any given moment, or do we create a fictional account around it? Or are we not even paying attention? Are our minds in a prison on lockdown, or are we just keeping ourselves busy so that we don't have to feel anything?

There are a thousand ways to deny reality. Lunatics like Hitler and other horrible human beings create completely extravagant, insane, and totally warped realities to deny the truth of their inner pain. It doesn't work. The pain will still rise to the surface. And when a person can deny it, even as it's rising to the surface, the feelings will begin to corrode him or her. Denial sets the base for a toxic mind and chemistry.

These are my theories. I'm sharing them with you because these theories have been extremely helpful to me and have led to big breakthroughs. Since the beginning of my recovery at age 15, I've needed to break through my walls of denial. That denial centered around the agony and pain that I experienced starting when I was a child.

At times I do everything in my power to prevent myself from feeling. I consider myself a pretty good human being—I'm not doing wacky, headline-worthy, sensational negative and destructive things. I'm really trying. Yet I have to climb over denial all the time. I make up stories for myself and I create false realities. But now I'm always aware that right around the corner of these false realities there are fragments of what were once called feelings. I have to face them if I want to reach my maximum capacity. And I do want to reach it. I'll be striving to do that for the rest of my life, even if I live to be 160.

I don't believe that we ever completely eradicate denial. There's a type of balance between truth, reality, and the fictions that we create that are based in denial. One thing you need to realize is that denial wasn't and isn't an entirely bad thing. When you had certain feelings in the past and you couldn't cope with them, thank God you had denial. Denial saved you. Say to yourself right now that you're grateful to have had the ability to have denial.

However, when we become adults, denial no longer serves us well. It holds us back from truly being free. Now, we must figure out exactly what denials we have about the things that we're doing in the present. When we admit that we're doing them, then we can change them if we want to. This is so because we're saying to ourselves, "Hey, this thing is happening and I don't like it. I don't need to do it. I have a choice. I can change if I want to."

I know this stuff sounds extremely corny, but it's true. The way to break through denial is to write down the entire journey of your life. Don't leave out the facts, because as you write the journey down you're going to see it right in front of you. You're going to see what you did in the past, and you're going to see what you are doing in the present.

When I was 15, I had to write down, "I am an alcoholic, and I am a pothead." Those things controlled me—I didn't control them—and I didn't want to do them anymore. And when I said to myself that I had those problems, then said it out loud to myself and others, and then wrote it down, I was finally ready to take the next step.

It wasn't as if there suddenly was a miraculous explosion of light just because I admitted the truth about myself. But until I admitted that something was happening and that I had a problem with it, I was completely unable to take any type of step to change it.

A long time ago when I used to talk about denial to people who were new to sobriety, I would give them a ridiculous example. I would repeatedly slap my head with my hand, and then I'd say, "Wow, this really hurts." The person watching me, knowing my sense of humor, would wait for a punchline. But I'd just keep slapping my head and saying, "This really hurts." Then I would say, "But I'm not doing it. You're doing it to me!" And then I would say, "It's not really even happening." After that I would say, "It's happening and it hurts." Next, I would say, "It doesn't hurt. I can do this forever. I'm tough—nothing hurts me!"

After that silly display, I'd pause and then be quiet for a few moments. Then I'd say, "This really hurts and I'm doing it. I don't like it, and I want to stop it. I can see my hand slapping myself in the face. It's me who's doing it. How do I stop doing it?"

You can apply this lesson to weight control, food addiction, and all other problem areas of your life. You can do so by writing. Ask yourself these questions: What are you doing? What negative behaviors do you have? What hurts you? Are you truly happy? Do you feel sadness? Are you stuck? Are you using drugs addictively? Are you using alcohol addictively? Are you using food addictively? Are you in an addictive, toxic relationship?

Ask yourself all of these questions, and be gentle with yourself. But don't run away, and don't be afraid. Realize this: You're strong and you're here. You're in this book right now. You're reading. That means that you have strength and that you have found something. It means that your journey has started and you are ready to move forward.

I suggest if you're alone that you start a breathing exercise while you're standing. Walk back and forth. Pace 10 feet one way, then pace 10 feet the other way. Rub your chest with your left hand in a downward circular motion to start to warm your chest plate.

While you're doing this, tell yourself that you're ready to heal and ready to move forward. Tell yourself that you have the courage to do it. Tell yourself that you will do it.

Be patient with yourself. Go slow. Keep this book near you. Keep it on the shelf. Keep it in your computer bag. Keep a copy in your car. If you need extra copies, I'll give you two for the price of three.

To truly quit our poor eating habits, the very first thing we have to do is admit to ourselves that we have a problem. This principle is adopted from the 12-step program of Alcoholics Anonymous, and it's a great one!

The admission of the problem gets the proverbial ball rolling. The first step to solving any problem in one's life is to first admit that the problem exists. This first step of admission can be applied to a drug addiction, to a food addiction, a sex addiction, a gambling addiction, or any other type of addiction.

Writing Exercise: Once we have admitted that we have a problem, we need to write something similar to the following in our journal:

"Oftentimes throughout my life I've become powerless over an obsession and an addictive behavior pattern. At times in my life I can get control. I can do so through my own higher power. The times that I lose control I am totally powerless. I am powerless over my addiction to overeating junk food, undereating healthy food, and all the other dietary mistakes that make me feel poorly. As a result of this powerlessness, I often feel as though my life is unmanageable."

We will have to surrender and surrender over and over again throughout our lives, especially if we feel tempted to relapse. We surrender by saying, "I am ready to let you go now. This thing I'm doing is causing me problems. When I let you go I will be liberated and I will feel happy." (Note: That language is my own; you can come up with another phrase that better suits you if you wish, as long as you are sincerely expressing the same thought and intent.)

"I wish to quit doing this thing." This is a new reality. If you are willing to say those words with sincerity, you are one very big step closer to overcoming your problem. It's a new reality to step into "I quit" instead of "I'm still doing" or the reality that most get stuck in: "I'm too scared to try to quit."

32. Behavior Patterns Trigger Poor Dietary Choices

The process of you developing your own dietary patterns must include that you detox your eyeballs and your taste buds from things that you've become so accustomed to that they've shaped the way that you look at reality. If tomorrow you let go of most of the things that you did that were bad for you, but did not replace them with healthy alternatives, you would go through terrible emotional pain. You would feel as if you were stumbling in space alone, and you would likely not be able to get your bearings. And if you weren't aware that this was happening, then you'd be setting yourself up for a toxic food relapse.

Poor eating habits and patterns such as toxic food relapses have very painful psychological ties. The process of recovery is one of discovery into our personal sources of pain and then working towards healing them.

Coming to a proper understanding of poor eating choices requires exploration of your own psychology and behavior patterns. In doing so, you would probably be best served if you were in therapy with someone who understood addiction recovery and who dealt with patients with various attachment disorders.

Early attachment disorders and anxiety are definitely at the heart of any addictive behavior patterns. It will be necessary to learn about those things. It will also be necessary to write in your journal about how you're going to cope with difficult emotions other than through unhealthy eating. This step must remain fluid; you should be working on this for the rest of your life.

I felt anxiety very quickly when I would talk about my childhood experiences. I came to realize that I needed to move slowly so that anxiety would not consume me and shut me down.

I want to reiterate here how difficult the mastery of food is for a food addict. Food is the substance of all life. It is connected to our most primal feelings. The first thing we are given to soothe our discomfort when we come into this world is food, in the form of mother's milk.

It is likely that we will all develop some type of association of comfort with food. It's also possible to associate a lot of discomfort with food. To master weight loss, it's absolutely crucial to master all of the emotions that are associated with overeating and other negative eating patterns.

What we often don't realize is that when we are overeating, undereating, or eating the wrong foods, it's connected to our concepts of consumerism. We use substances to change the way we feel about reality. This comes from a modern mindset, in which it feels difficult for us to be in the moment; we almost always feel that we need to change something. **We have to work extremely hard to be focused and present.**

We learn as we grow up that food can change our chemistry and that it's available at all times. It then becomes very difficult when we reach a certain point to learn how to listen to the body. The body gives us very subtle signals about how it feels, but we can suffocate those signals over time.

Weight loss is not about cutting calories—it never was. Neither is it about exercising like a lunatic and burning calories in order to watch the pounds melt away.

• •

Weight loss is about losing the weight of certain behaviors. We need to gain conscious contact with our body again. Physical weight loss, therefore, is about peeling away the layers that insulate us from the physical experience of being in the body.

• •

We eat when we're anxious. We eat when we're happy. We eat when we're sad. We eat when we're angry. We eat when we're bored. We eat to transition from one thing to the next. We eat because someone told us it was time to. We eat to be social.

• •

But what we really need to do is to eat because we are hungry. We need to eat to nourish the body. We need to eat to replenish components from food that our bodies are losing on a daily basis.

• •

Then, one might argue, shouldn't eating be a chance for people to come together, socialize and enjoy each other? While that's an understandable personal preference, consider that that type of behavior can become a trap if it's left unchecked.

It's possible that your health is at risk because of eating patterns, and a big shift is required. Certainly eat when you're hungry (to a reasonable degree), eat with your partner, and eat with your family. But be aware if you are eating out of sequence for the purpose of changing your feelings.

Writing Exercise: Explore your associations with food as far back as you can remember. Does anxiety impact your overeating?

33. The Relationship Between Physical Exercise and Happiness

Most certainly, exercise is crucial to overall health. (I will cover more on the topic of exercise in Part Five of this book.) You don't need to beat your body into the ground seven days a week to be happy. Doing so could become a compulsion; a compulsion such that your body signals to you that something is wrong because it's not completely exhausted.

Exercising in this way is detrimental to the body. We need to work the body until it is just the right amount of tired. In going past a reasonable limit, we are not just exhausting the body but exhausting the mind as well.

That doesn't mean you shouldn't love your exercise, work out, and push yourself hard when you're young and strong. Just make sure that you understand what your intentions are: Really be honest with yourself.

You may be exercising in excess because of a lack of self-love—because you don't like yourself if you feel fat.

Or maybe you're judging yourself harshly because you ate a cookie: Then you feel that you have to work out until you are completely exhausted and positive that the cookie calories have been burned off.

Improper motivation and action in exercise are examples of how not dealing with emotional and psychological issues in appropriate ways relate to weight control problems. It's very important to be aware of the things that motivate and drive you as you pursue effective, long-term weight loss.

If you need to work out excessively to feel comfortable in your own body, then you should change your intention. Don't say to yourself, "I'm doing this to burn calories and take that extra one inch off my waist." Instead, change your intention, so that you can say, "Strong exercise makes me feel great—it gives me a clear perspective and it makes me happy."

Intention is crucial. So are quite a number of other psychological factors, which will be explained in some detail in this book.

Exercising regularly will have a positive effect on your mood, and subsequently on your desire to remain engaged in a healthy diet and lifestyle. We need to move our bodies regularly, and we need the chemicals that exercise produces—cortisol and endorphins.

Writing Exercise: What is your motivation behind exercise? Is it solely vanity-based, or do you enjoy the physical feeling of it?

34. Stop Saying Unkind Things to Yourself

All people, and in particular us westerners, have a tendency to look at ourselves in our mirrors and judge ourselves—either too kindly or too harshly. We need to consider why that's the case. When did that start? With the invention of mirrors? Or with the invention of the eating of junk food, overeating, and consuming too many debaucherous foods?

(I'm coining the nonexistent word "debaucherous" in this comment. I could use the terms overindulgent foods, decadent foods, or treats. But I don't think any of them are strong enough words to communicate the destructive potential of these particular food products.)

A major distraction from the focus of your success with diet is beating yourself up when you see yourself in the mirror. You might as well go by the mirror one last time and say, "Man, am I ugly or what? I am ugly!" Now that you've done that, you can move on and focus on all of the true things that matter.

Think of all of the things that really make your life amazing. If you are utterly gorgeous, blessings and thank you for letting us see you. If you are just regular like most people, that's a blessing too. You have an endless number of enviable qualities worth focusing on. They are your superpowers.

Stop focusing on your presumed weakness(es). Break the obsession. It's pointless and all-consuming. Focus first on what your heart is made of. How well do you love? How happy can you be? How happy can you make others? Get yourself in focus by concentrating on something other than what you see as your weakness. It may take a lot of practice, but you need to do it.

Writing Exercise: What do you see in the mirror? How does it impact the way you eat?

It seems as if we needed mirrors to look at ourselves because we started learning how to feel what our bodies felt like—whether or not they felt full or uncomfortable.

Does it feel painful, both emotionally and physically, to not be in our ideal bodies? We should define what an ideal body is, because everyone has a different concept of what ideal is.

For the purposes of discussion about the subject, we need to create a baseline. And we cannot separate physical health from emotional health, because the two are combined; the two deeply affect each other.

One concept is simple. Specifically, putting food in your mouth represents many things at different times of your life, and at different times of the day, eating consists of many symbolic gestures. The most profound one is that eating is a means of reconnecting to the umbilical cord.

I have a theory, which is as follows: By putting food into your mouth, you are creating a symbolic cord or connection from the outside world to your hunger, from your stomach to your sense of safety with your mother. It's no wonder that we like to eat or even just hold things that look like food—it's a symbolic gesture that reconnects us to the umbilical cord. Even though it's not literal and even though it's subconscious, it still has significant meaning and feels very good.

But there are other meanings that are significant as well. Sometimes we can even feel weightless when we feel hunger. So we fuel ourselves, but that doesn't really do the trick. It gives us a temporary feeling of being glued to the earth because we are weighted down by food and beverages.

• •

Human beings, like all species of animals, have an engineered program within our design regarding how we're supposed to eat as a species. It's specific, and it encompasses types of foods, quantities of food, and optimal times of day to eat. We also have it recorded in our superconscious mind—eating food entails rituals and customs.

• •

But what if a person feels very disconnected from their primeval and natural ways of eating? What if our childhoods and early disruptions caused us to look at food in a way that is harmful to ourselves?

If we look at food the wrong way and let it control our eating practices over a lifetime, should that behavior be considered food addiction? Bad eating habits? Pathological behavior? Or innocent unconsciousness? Is destructive eating a sign of emotional problems? Or is it just habituation formed by regular, constantly-learned bad habits? It's important to answer those particular questions before we can really start to change things.

One thing is certain: Adults can be extremely focused on any subject if they choose to be, and they can have an incredible capacity to be honest with themselves about what they do and feel.

I speak from experience when I say that my relationship with food started off as a bit of a struggle. I got control of it when I was young and I worked very hard my whole life to maintain a specific type of diet. I became very mindful of my own tendencies and hyper-focused on the tendencies of some family members who were obese. They overate for many different emotional reasons and in ways that they admitted were destructive.

••

People should think of their diets in a way that extends beyond the physical benefits. They can think about their diets in terms of how those diets will affect their moods, emotions, spirituality, and more. The foods you eat should help you realize and understand your place in the universe. Food can have a gigantic impact on your emotional well-being.

••

For example, you may have grown up in a family which ate together harmoniously on Friday through Sunday nights, where each member knew that they were loved and accepted at the family dinner table. Even if the foods eaten were full of heavy starches and meat sauces, those particular foods conjured up the same happy feelings when the same foods were eaten later in life. Those foods, despite being harmful to their health, still had a positive impact on their emotional well-being.

• •

The trick in life is to align emotional well-being with foods that are healthy—not just for the human body but for the planet as well. Then, when one eats, he or she can both nourish their body and feel a greater connection to Mother Earth.

• •

Writing Exercise: What were your family eating experiences like throughout your life? What emotions does it conjure up for you when you think about being at the dinner table, especially at holidays and evening meals? If there were no real patterns of being together at evening mealtimes, how did that affect you?

35. About Childhood Trauma

People with exceedingly analytical minds have a problem at times. They can become so focused on particular issues that they are pondering that they have difficulty with intellectually living in the present moment. All of us at certain times in life can find ourselves terrified of the future, stuck in the past, or overwhelmed by all of the fart bubbles constantly popping into our heads.

But the goal is to not be hindered from living in the here and now when such thoughts occur. The ultimate goal of the psychological work that you are involving yourself with in this health-related endeavor is to develop a "steel mind." You want to bring yourself to a level of consciousness that enables you to live moment to moment.

The journey of recovery does involve taking periodic pauses and stepping backward to think about some of the things that happened to you in the past. The purpose of doing so is to bring up the emotions so that you can let them move through you and subsequently be cleared. You should look back at painful moments so that you can deal with them and move on. But you shouldn't live in those places and times.

Painful moments don't just dissipate on their own. Time does not heal all wounds—some wounds can stay with us forever. So it's critically important that we understand that there's no danger in spending a little bit of time revisiting the past for the purpose of setting ourselves free from the negative effects of it.

It's important that you don't try to find every possible uncomfortable or disturbing moment from the past. It's equally as important that you recognize critical things that happened to you that caused you to establish negative lifestyle patterns. Doing so is foundational to the healing work that you are taking on.

Our overall emotional well-being must be a high priority. This relates not only to weight control issues, but to physical and mental well-being as it touches all aspects of our life. That being the case, understanding and dealing with childhood trauma is crucial.

We must understand that we were damaged by our early experiences and that eating poorly has become our ill-formed defense. Turning to addictive patterns to numb and offset feelings is an unsatisfactory psychological mechanism. The bad feelings pile up and make us mentally unwell, and we subsequently act out in any way that we can in order to feel better.

In this day and age we spend enormous amounts of emotional energy and time trying to liberate ourselves from the past difficulties of our lives. Of course there have been beautiful experiences in the lives of most everyone; marriages, children, business successes, etc. But it's a problem that these things have been conditions that brought us happiness. The feeling of joy about just being alive should be our only condition for happiness.

Most of us had that joy when we were children, but we lost it. Now we have to set out to recover it. Most of us think of recovery (e.g., 12-step recovery) in terms of recovering from the damage that our addictions have caused us. But recovery should be thought of not only in terms of recovering from something negative or damaging. Recovery should also be thought of as the attempt to regain something positive.

That positive thing is usually something a little bit different for every person. As an example, the desperate drunk is trying to recover the ability to live happily and productively when sober. Speaking for myself, I'm trying to recover the tremendous joy I had from just being a child, being able to feel and express my feelings, desiring to explore the world, experience things, and find laughter.

The simple joys of childhood are what a great many people are trying to recover. But in addition to childhood joy, I'm trying to recover the ability to just live in the moment and not drift into unproductive thought processes or obsessions. I don't want to constantly be lost in the past or be thinking anxiously about the future. I want to be here, in the present, with my feet on the ground, looking at the trees, taking in deep breaths, and feeling the pleasant sensations of the moment.

Yet in childhood we also experienced uncomfortable and traumatic things. We learned to drift away from certain moments of that time because those particular moments were uncomfortable. When we live in the past we focus a lot on moments of sadness and feelings of loss and desperation. And even if the past was beautiful, if we compare it to a present moment then we may be disappointed that the present moment is not as beautiful.

At this point you may find some of these reflections to be a bit disturbing. But it is crucial to realize that unhealthy psychological and emotional patterns must be overcome if you're seeking to achieve healthy dietary patterns in general and permanent weight loss in particular. Achieving those goals is the proverbial "light at the end of the tunnel."

36. Addressing Childhood Trauma and Emotional Issues

Some believe that addictions are just accidents that people fall into, and they need only to rid themselves of the addictions to get back to normal. This is not correct. I will venture to say that every human being that has an addiction also has attachment disorders, anxiety, and experiences with trauma (most likely in childhood).

The word "trauma" sounds imposing and somewhat scary. It sounds as if it's referring to something frightening, such as watching someone have their arm severed in a car accident. Yet far less dramatic things can also be defined as traumas. Children are traumatized very easily because they're naïve and they don't understand what's happening at times. They interpret things that you and I might laugh at as being threats to their survival.

If children experience deprivation from emotional needs, the effects can be traumatic. An example might be that of a child who didn't get enough consistent attention from a father who was constantly working. The child might have developed deep anxieties as a result. Later in life, he or she may have developed addictions to help cope with the unmet longing.

••

In order to beat food addictions, it's necessary to identify the unmet emotional needs in your life and take steps to overcome them.

••

Doing so will take work, and the work may be difficult. But the definition of what the work itself entails is simple. The work consists of doing the following things:

- ► Discovering what traumatic events or patterns happened to you as a child through talking and writing about them ("getting them out on the table," so to speak).
- ► Calling siblings, parents, and close friends who witnessed your childhood to help fill in the blanks regarding what you don't remember or what you perceived incorrectly.
- ► Finding a safe place to talk about the events and issues.
- ► Being willing to feel some very scary emotions.
- ► Possibly getting angry and crying.
- ► Slowly letting those trapped emotions evaporate.

Dealing with emotions connected to traumatic experiences coupled with adapting new lifestyle habits will enable you to master any addiction.

It is absolutely critical to master the feelings that we have trapped inside of us from the past. If we don't do so, we are condemned to continue to consciously or unconsciously use defense mechanisms and systems that are designed to protect us from feelings caused by trauma.

••

We act out in our adult behavior to suppress the anxiety and the negative emotions connected to what happened to us when we were kids. If we want to stop the behaviors forever, we have to do two things: We have to heal any unhealed trauma, and we have to create new behavior patterns.

••

Symptoms of being trapped in our defense mechanisms include eating disorders, depression, difficult to manage anxiety, relationship problems, unhappiness, and many, many other things. The list is virtually endless.

••

Childhood experiences, particularly the traumatic ones, absolutely must be looked at, faced up to, and overcome.

••

You may have very thick walls of denial or a total lack of memory about various childhood experiences that need to be examined.

One of the most common psychological characteristics that adults have is that they have it in their heads that they need to protect their parents at all costs from any negative words. This is also a defense mechanism.

We protect our parents selfishly as a lifetime habit. It's not because of biblical obligations; it's because somewhere deep in our minds we associate our survival with our parents being superheroes and great people. If we face up to the fact that they may have made a lot of mistakes, then the walls of protection around our trauma start to crumble. We are left with feelings of depression and loss, and those feelings can be very frightening.

It might be the case that you don't suffer from any particular physical or mental afflictions. But that is not the case with most people. The majority of us need to confront the feelings that have wounded us. This begins with expressing those emotions in the presence of others.

37. Identify Difficult Emotional Checkpoints That Lead to Negative Behavior

I have found the following practice to be very helpful, and I strongly recommend it. Check in two or three times daily with yourself, asking "How do I feel?," and "What am I craving?"

► Sweet craving	► Full feeling
► Empty feeling	► Anxiety
► Creative	► Angry
► Resentful	► Energetic
► Bored	► Active
► Pensive	► Lonely
► Need touch	► Need solitude
► Hungry	► Starving
► Fearful	► Sexual

These are a few of the checkpoints to identify before eating. Put a name to what you feel on a deeper level during the day.

Sometimes I check in with myself at 12 noon and I'm elated. At 2 PM I feel resentful about something someone said to me. I might feel triggered to think about a deeper wound. I am unsettled. Then, I am eating. How does this feeling affect what I decide to eat?

An exercise that I have stuck with over the years is to lay quietly as I am waking, eyes closed, and try to associate one or two words with how it feels in my body and how it feels in my mind. Today I awoke and thought, "I feel tired and I feel sad about something." I could not trace the sadness to anything. I think I was just tired. So I was able to say to myself, "You are tired, not sad. Go slow and do something to inspire yourself." I followed my wake-up routine and then immediately started writing, "It's afternoon and I am writing this and I feel relaxed and productive. I am tired from my workout yesterday. I am glad I did it. I need to eat for success today. I need to drink a lot of water. I need a big salad. I want a super ripe banana."

I am sharing this with you so that you can understand my process. This type of writing is a way that I stay very connected with myself and I can address my sensations and thoughts before they get way ahead of me, after which I may react or act out negatively. It's extremely important to me to **document my feelings in writing.**

38. Feel Your Feelings

Human beings are sensing and feeling creatures. We have our five senses: sight, hearing, taste, touch, and smell. We also have our internal emotions/feelings. What feelings are is much harder to explain than the basic five senses. The feelings are linked to the five senses and also to our thought processes.

The most pervasive feeling for an addicted person is fear. Pervasive fear is also known as anxiety. Adults who survived mild to severe trauma and neglect as children will likely live with anxieties that originated in childhood for their entire lives. They may or may not be aware of the presence of that anxiety.

We live with these anxieties, and they affect us until we find a way to unravel them and be free of them. The anxieties will be experienced in a variety of ways, but pervasive anxiety is a particularly painful physical and emotional experience.

We seek relief from this pain and distress by either talking about it—actually feeling the feelings behind the anxiety—or by repressing the feelings and the anxiety. If we repress them, it means that we hold them down by acting out. We can find countless ways to act out, including food addictions and behaviors to repress the feelings and the anxiety that follows.

The only way to face anxiety is to first admit that it exists. If we have anxiety, it must be linked to a feeling that caused fear at a different time in life. In our childhoods, we may not have been able to express our fears or to resolve them. This is the nature of the dysfunctional childhood. This is the common trauma in the dysfunctional childhood—not being allowed to have feelings or to express them.

You might remember your childhood as being very gentle and passive with very present and complete parents. But if you have addictions as a grown-up, it's likely that something very negative occurred during that time. Everything might have been close to perfect in your childhood. However, if you weren't able to identify your feelings and express them, then that was dysfunction.

And of course most of us experienced things that were much worse than just not being able to have our feelings. Many of us were hit, many of us did not get the attention we needed, and many of us were programmed with faulty messages regarding our very existence. Some of us were exposed to things too early, and we sadly had to witness our own parents' internal suffering.

If your primary caregivers did these things to you, it means that they likely went through similar experiences during their childhoods. These problems get passed down from generation to generation, the same way that eye color and skin color do. The cycle of such mistreatment and mild to severe abuse will never end until people confront the problem.

The problem is that one of the survival mechanisms that we build in our mind is that of pure denial. And the simple fact is that if you had a wonderful childhood you would not be addicted to anything. I dare any psychologist or philosopher to prove me wrong: That's my one challenge to anyone in this field.

The way to move through anxiety, which is the ultimate causation for addiction, is to work through it. It's difficult to do that when we're awake and totally alert sitting in the therapist's chair. Our defenses and distractions are really strong. We need to be in a relaxed yet very awake state. (That's why it's difficult to do meditation work while laying in bed; you're likely to fall asleep.)

The beginning portion of anxiety discovery is to sit somewhere quiet facing the ocean, or to lay in the 'dead body pose' in the living room. When I do so, I like to play New Age frequency sound wave music that I find on YouTube; music with lyrics is too distracting for me to explore my mind. I do deep breathing exercises while laying on my back, and I very quickly find an anxiety that lingers.

I try to pick up that anxiety in my mind and follow it to its source as I can remember it. Then I tell myself, "Right now, as an adult, I'm anxious because of "blank."" Then I go from that source and try to link it to an earlier source, and I keep tracing it. While I'm tracing it I'm breathing and I'm aware of my breath.

I usually find something that links me to some memories in my early adult life, my teenage years, or to some point in my childhood. When I get to my childhood, oftentimes I cannot find an emotion. I just have a few memories and perhaps a couple of intellectual thoughts about them, but I can't feel them yet. I have to write those memories down, and then I have to guess how I think a normal person would feel if that experience happened to them. Then I have to ask myself, "Where are those feelings? Why don't I feel anything about that situation that happened?"

And that's where the work begins. There's a simple solution: It's not going to take me a week to get over the fact that my mom had a severe rage outburst at me when I was very little and slapped and punched me because she couldn't deal with her feelings of frustration. I was taught at that moment that I was a bad child. The safety and the trust a child should have with a mother was lost. I can't feel anything about that—I'm numb.

But then I realize that I'm supposed to be feeling something about it. Because 45 years later I have anxieties about things and addictions that keep flaring up. For me, the association between my childhood and my adult behavior then becomes clear.

The heart of your recovery work will be the time that you spend identifying childhood experiences and finding your feelings. You then eventually get to the point where you can feel them, where you can get angry, cry, go deeper, and grieve.

Then what happens? Those feelings pass! Over time, we may have to go through those exercises several times until we get to a place where the energy is dispersed. At that point we let go of it naturally, not just because we made a decision to let go of it. We let go of it in the way that feelings are actually processed.

We don't let go of a feeling intellectually by saying to ourselves, "Well, I've learned to forgive!" We let go of feelings by feeling them. If we don't feel them, then they just stay in our body.

If they stay in our body, they will influence the way that we think. If they were terrifying experiences or very painful experiences, we built up defenses to avoid feeling the terror or pain again.

Behaving in that way becomes an obsession: We are obsessed with our survival and our protection. That obsession is also physically painful. It drives us crazy: There's a subtle torment behind addictions, and we're trying to get it out. The only way to get it out is to realize it, explore it, find all of it, understand it, feel it, and then make needed corrections in behavior.

It's not something that is easily done on your own. You should have expert guidance from either a professional or some type of a healer who can guide you through this. The work is vitally important: It will lead you to true knowledge of self and freedom from addiction and suffering.

The healing process is more complex than the summary of it that I've described. That is why it takes time. In the meantime, you should still be on your path to arrest addictive behavior. And you need to realize that there will always be stressful situations in your adult life, and those experiences will conjure up anxiety.

Not everything you feel today has to be linked to the time that you didn't get a balloon at a birthday party, cried, and then got slapped across the face. But the human brain works in such a way that it makes associations with things like that: If something happens to us as grownups, we immediately make an association to what it feels like that was familiar to a memory from another point in life.

The liberation from addictive behavior does not have to come when you are at the final stages of emotional healing from all the traumas and experiences of your childhood. You don't have to wait 10 years to stop eating chocolate cake at 2 o'clock in the morning. Just by engaging in this new process of tracing today's feelings back to earlier experiences, and just by giving yourself the permission to feel old repressed feelings, you have begun your journey. And you should be excited about that.

When we find a solution to our anxiety, there's hope. The solution is to feel the feelings that caused the anxiety in the first place. When we begin the journey of feeling again, anything could happen. We may feel more anxious for a while before we can feel relieved. Don't be dissuaded by periods of confusion when you can't drop old feelings.

You might move through sadness and then through a sense of loss. You can go back and forth between anger and forgiveness, then back to denial of what happened in your childhood, then back to anger, forgiveness, depression, and so on. This is the emotional recovery aspect of the work. As we get better at it, we will be able to cope with those feelings and still lead a normal life.

By normal I mean that you will experience ups and downs and difficulties in life forever, but you won't have to behave self-destructively as a result. It's going to take time to work on all of these internal emotional problems that have their origins in your early life. The amount of time will vary from one individual to another.

But you can't rush these healing processes. Your subconscious mind won't let you. This is why it's highly advisable that a person seeks counseling to accelerate the process and make sure that it stays on course.

You may need help along the way to figure out certain aspects of the logic of your emotional recovery. You may need guidance to understand what you're feeling. This is so because when difficult emotions come up, they're surrounded by all kinds of conflicting emotions at the same time. That gets confusing—but this is what the work entails. It's very difficult for some. But it's much more difficult to live your life not doing this work and instead remain caught up in the maze of addictive cycles.

As you pursue healing by doing the appropriate work related to dealing with your feelings, it's crucial that you verbally express emotions to the appropriate support people. Such people include therapists, loved ones, best friends, and others that you feel safe around and can trust. You must maintain this process until the day you die.

• •

I very strongly suggest that you talk about the new behavior that you want to achieve and discuss your feelings with others, starting today. Rather than just contemplating thoughts regarding desired/undesired behavior and uncomfortable feelings, it is important for your growth that you talk about them.

• •

By doing so, your expression of emotions will bring the energy of the experience out from repression within and into the external world. This will transform what's internal and not real yet into something external and tangible that can then be accessed and healed.

This may seem too simple and/or very radical as a technique to approaching weight loss, but it is a necessary procedure. An explanation of why this is so requires consideration of some physical and psychological principles pertaining to emotions.

Writing Exercise: Who can I talk to? Do I have enough people to talk to? If I don't, where will I find more people to talk to? If need be, how can I find a more robust support group? Create solutions in your writing.

39. Bodily Processing of Emotions

The body uses certain mechanical processes to remove its toxic materials. For example, perspiration, urination, and defecation all remove carbonic acid (a byproduct of cellular metabolism) from the blood so that life-giving oxygen can get in.

Similarly, our body uses certain mechanical processes when we experience feelings. When we feel deep sadness we cry. We make different facial expressions and/or change our body language depending on how we feel. When we're amused we make noises with laughter. Sometimes we move our bodies in certain ways because we're having particular feelings. We express emotions in these ways and others.

But during or after experiencing trauma we're usually very hesitant to express our feelings about it. This is especially the case concerning trauma in early childhood and/or trauma that occurred in our family of origin. We witnessed and experienced things that were painful, difficult, or abusive.

We feel incredibly powerful emotions, but we don't necessarily feel safe to express them. We learn to shut down our crying and hold our anger in. An entire defense system is built around shutting down emotions to protect ourselves from the difficulty of them. Both children and adults, but especially children, need encouragement, explanations, and help in learning how to describe their feelings and process them.

As I mentioned before, one of the great mechanisms for releasing emotions is to communicate them through language by speaking with another human being. We are absolutely designed for that particular process, but sometimes we may not be able to find or express our feelings as we try to recover in life.

However, just passively thinking about your own particular traumas may not be enough to discover what you need to about what happened in your life.

Writing Exercise: Write about what experiences you had and what feelings about them may be trapped inside of you. Write specifically on the worst things that have happened in your life: This is a key exercise to bring you to self-knowledge.

Feelings can dissipate over time, but they can also latch their way into your thinking and make you become stuck in harmful physical and emotional behaviors, sometimes for your entire life. Your feelings will affect the way you think and they will affect the way you respond and react to situations going forward.

You have to learn to express your trapped emotions, and you have to understand their sources. You must learn to understand the situations that caused them, particularly the situations that were traumatic.

Some people are terrified to share their emotions. A person asked to talk about feelings with a therapist might freeze at the idea because he or she wouldn't know what to expect. Even extremely tough people may have deep, dark fears that if they experience certain emotions then they'll die. This is related to things that happened to them during their childhoods.

Many developed an unhealthy belief system from early childhood about what it means to feel. Too many children were told to be quiet at inappropriate times. Some children who complained and cried were told by their parents things such as, "Stop crying or I'll give you something to really cry about." They were threatened. So, for many, the process of feeling became corrupted.

Our entire journey in life is a thought process. We need to learn new things. We have to teach ourselves things, and we need to overcome barriers to moving forward as they present themselves in the form of improper handling of our own thoughts and emotions.

40. Repressing Emotions Can Make Us Physically and Emotionally Sick

We have got to get the historical emotions that are locked away in the safe zones of our mind out. If we don't, they will eventually intoxicate the body with their physical altering capabilities. But during or after experiencing trauma we're usually very hesitant to express our feelings.

This is especially true of trauma in early childhood and/or trauma that occurred in our family of origin. When we witness and experience things that are painful, difficult, or abusive, we feel incredibly powerful emotions, but we don't usually feel safe expressing them.

We hold our anger in and shut down our crying. **Our mind has a complex defense system that is built around shutting down emotions to protect ourselves from the difficulty of dealing with them.**

For both children and adults, one of the great mechanisms for releasing emotions is to communicate them by speaking with another person (or group of people). We are absolutely designed for doing so. But in trying to recover in life we may have difficulty finding or expressing our feelings.

••

Just thinking about your own particular traumas usually isn't nearly enough to discover what you need to about your unpleasant emotional experiences in life. You need to understand and analyze those experiences and the feelings about them that are trapped inside of you.

••

Sometimes feelings dissipate over time. But very often—likely more often than not—they find their way into your thinking patterns. Sometimes they make you become stuck in harmful behaviors, both physical and emotional, and sometimes for your whole life. The feelings will affect how you respond and react to situations going forward. We have to learn to express our trapped emotions, and we have to understand their sources—the situations that caused them.

41. Therapy Is Important

As you pursue good physical health, you must simultaneously pursue good mental health. It is absolutely crucial to get in touch with your feelings and learn how to deal with them. And again, the best way of doing so is to talk with and listen to others.

In this information age you can browse the internet to find online groups, brick and mortar real people groups, all different types of groups that you can participate in to talk to and listen to live people discussing feelings.

This is how we make positive progress with our emotions; this is where we begin to develop the tools to arrest the dysfunctional behaviors, dietary and otherwise, that we wish to rid ourselves of. And this is what therapy is all about.

Should you be in some type of therapy? The answer is always a resounding yes. But it's often not easy for a person to find therapy at an affordable price. The majority of people I know avoid therapy completely because of its cost. Some people I know avoid it regardless of its cost because they just don't want to spend money on such an activity. And some don't know of effective alternatives to expensive therapy. But there are such alternatives available.

The most effective type of therapy is a group setting facilitated by a mental health care professional. It's desirable for a number of reasons. For one thing, the cost will be considerably less than that of sessions with an individual private therapist.

Also, the group dynamic is important and helpful. People around you will bring up feelings that you have a hard time getting in touch with. When they talk about themselves, you will hear things that bring up anger, sadness, frustration, and other emotions. You will need to learn how to deal with these emotions as you pursue your recovery from food addiction.

Another good thing about group therapy is that you have a number of people to project your life onto rather than just one therapist. The additional feedback will be helpful. My opinion, based on personal experience and much study on the matter, is that group therapy is often more effective than multiple one-on-one sessions with a therapist.

Most group therapy environments aren't sessions focused on single topics. Usually you meet once per week in the same place, and a therapist will be present along with other individuals like yourself who are seeking to overcome various things. A ballpark price (at the time of this writing) for a one- or two-hour session might be around two silver coins or five chickens. Your turn to speak would come, and at that point you would talk about your addictions or whatever was trapped in your head.

There are exceptions to unfocused group therapy sessions. Certain matters are best discussed in highly specialized groups: These include groups that are tailored to sexual abuse survivors or people overcome with grief over the death of a loved one. In such cases it's preferable to be among those connected by the same types of troubling events.

At this point in the book we will move from psychological considerations regarding unhealthy eating to information about improving your dietary choices and practices. You will find this information to be interesting, somewhat challenging, and extremely beneficial if you choose to put it into practice.

Consider that the mind is an extraordinarily complex machine. Even with the unbelievable technological advances and the breakthroughs that we've had in scientific discoveries, we still know so little about how the mind and the body function. I believe that although humanity is in the dark ages when it comes to knowledge of the body, we're still doing pretty good.

One day all of the different fields of science will come together and have an A+ system to approach all aspects of healing. Right now, I think humanity gets a C minus. Even in the future when we get our A- and we know lots of stuff that we don't know today, I still believe that a human being would have to live 600 years to resolve all of his or her character defects and other problems.

I think that after 600 years you'd be able to get all of your childhood issues resolved, you'd be able to get rid of all your fears, you'd live moment to moment, and you'd have a clear connection to all of the knowledge in the universe. You are a work in progress. Unlike building a structure that has a foundation, a beginning, and an end to its construction, humanity will always be a work in progress: There is no ending lesson, except the journey from dying to death.

Say something positive to yourself on a daily basis—something that communicates that you are trying and that you know that you are on a positive journey towards your healing. This will have a profound impact on your anxiety levels.

That's been the case with me as I've been in the process of writing this book. I started monitoring when anxieties of any kind would come up within me. When they did, the first thing I would say to myself was, "I am on the positive side of my journey. My life, the world, and everything in it is positive. I choose to see it that way."

42. A Story Illustration

Please consider the following account of an interaction I had with someone many years ago:

One night a friend and I were talking on the phone. Toward the end of the conversation he asked me a question about himself. He asked me if I thought that at any point in his life that he would ever become a vegan and also stop drinking alcohol. (He was admitting that he was a heavy wine drinker.)

My answer to him was that there's no way that I could know what path he will eventually be on. I said that the fact that he was asking that question meant that there were two things on his mind: That veganism sparked his interest, and that he thought that wine drinking was a dependency problem for him.

I asked him if he was aware of whether or not he had a good or bad childhood. He replied that he thought it was pretty good. I also asked him if he thought that he had addictive behaviors or anxiety that prevented him from getting the maximum enjoyment out of life.

He said yes to both. I told him that the anxiety and addictive behaviors didn't match with the scenario that his childhood was pretty good. It was the right moment for me to ask him to recall the worst experience of his childhood.

He proceeded to tell me about one day when he was about eight and was sitting at the dinner table. His mother got angry about something (he couldn't remember what), came into the dining room, and grabbed his and his older sister's hair. She began to pull his hair so hard it felt as if it would rip out of his head.

He didn't have much detail after that. I quietly said to him that it sounds like your childhood was filled with trauma.

It sounds like that moment was humiliating, disgraceful, and frightening.

I then asked him if it was an isolated incident or if there had been others like it. He was quiet for a moment and then said his childhood was filled with incidents like that. Then he told me how he just learned to cope with the difficulties, survive, and always find ways to make the best of things.

I told him that his ability to cope, survive, and be such a productive member of society was a real testament to his true nature. I asked him to imagine how amazing his life would become if he was free of all of the encumbrances and interferences of a traumatic childhood.

I told him that he was missing the big picture. The big picture was that he was trapped in a loop. He suffered terrible abuse as a child. He had to shut down his emotions and alter his perception of the truth in order to survive. He created a series of defensive behaviors that he carries with him in his adult life. But the underlying feelings are still there, and they're still vibrating.

Anxieties are reactions to traumatic events. And addictive behaviors are coping mechanisms that actually do bring relief for a time. For a time, eating poorly, drinking too much, cigarette smoking, compulsive working, always having to be on the move, and other such things all serve a function. They get us through traumatic events, enabling our survival. But then we metaphorically move through life with a limp. We have all kinds of emotional disadvantages that prevent us from being the best versions of ourselves that we could be.

After coming to admission about just one event in his childhood he was able to see a clear picture. That one admission about something that happened is going to shape and change him forever. It may take him another 30 years for him to make the necessary changes to continue with deep diving emotional work. Or it may only take him 25 minutes.

43. Peoples' Motivations for Going on Diets

I spent close to 10 years at Juice Press involving myself in other people's dietary behavior. I learned a lot about how people in New York City feel about food. I know what their beliefs systems are, and I can make a lot of anecdotal statements about the general ideas and notions that people have about their diets.

One of the first groups of people I observed consisted of those who were healthy but who wanted to get more in shape. So their idea of a diet was just to reduce the number of calories they were consuming. The only thing they wanted to change in their lifestyle eating patterns was to eat less for a period of time until they reached their goals. This required discipline and motivation.

The next group of people that I observed consisted of those who struggled with weight for many years. Many had tried every possible diet program, including calorie restriction and working out more, but somehow or other they ended up back in an undesirable place. The lifestyle that we offered at Juice Press was just the latest and greatest fad to them, and many people just wanted to try out all the fads that they became aware of.

The last group of people that I observed consisted of those who came to Juice Press seeking salvation because they had some type of illness. Whether it was cancer, irritable bowel syndrome, or one of many other serious maladies, they were motivated by the desire to get better and not necessarily by their desire to drop weight.

44. The Error of Seeking Dietary Advice

Some experts simply give bad advice. Some books have some good information but also contain dietary mistakes at the heart of what the content teaches. Beware of being led to the less-than-optimal diet.

Many who are considering dietary changes come to knowledgeable people asking for dietary advice. But they often come with their own expectations about what they will be told and how much leeway they will be given in terms of taking that advice.

The metaphor I use to describe how I talk to people about getting help from someone like me is as follows: Imagine that you went to do a tandem skydive for the first time; you went to jump out of an airplane with a master skydiver and you had never jumped before.

Imagine that upon meeting the tandem jumpmaster you give him instructions on what you want the skydive procedures to be. You tell him how your harness should go on, at what altitude to open the parachute, and then once under a parachute you tell him how to navigate the parachute back to the landing area.

Another metaphor pertains to martial arts training. You finally get around to joining that Thai Boxing gym in New York. You go there for the first session and tell the instructor how you want to learn to throw a good right-handed punch. You then tell the Thai Boxing instructor how a kick should be blocked. This of course would be completely ludicrous.

In both examples I am reminded of how people seek help with nutrition and their diets. Most people know absolutely nothing about food. They know what it tastes like and they have some notions about what is good for them and what isn't. When they're trying to help themselves and they come to somebody who has understanding and takes time to explain things to them, they become the teacher and resist. It's as if they do this because they don't like what's being told to them.

Being more specific about how this works regarding diet, you have to change your patterns and habits that have built up over a long time. Your head is filled with misinformation and even lies about food and concepts that have been passed down to you from generation to generation.

45. Mealtimes and Misconceptions

In the western world we have a tendency to eat too many meals as a customary pattern. Two primary meals are generally needed by our bodies, but three is the norm for most people and that's OK.

The custom is somewhat in keeping with how we break up our day. The daytime (for most of us) is a time to be in action—working, playing, and discovering. Energy is needed, so it's appropriate to eat during the day.

We are optimally designed to eat fresh fruit early in the morning. As you begin your new diet, be sure to have a good selection of fresh fruits that are compatible with each other. Keep in mind that nutrients are not just physical substances, but entities that provide information to systems in your body. They not only provide vital compounds and sustenance, but they also transmit energy to our electrical system, our digestive system, our bloodstream, and our consciousness.

Many traditional breakfast items are in effect "dead foods." Although they provide calories and some nutrients, they are surprisingly devoid of many critical nutrients.

Such foods include overcooked greens, fried eggs, and breakfast meats such as bacon. The satisfaction that we feel after eating them is deceptive.

Eating during the day provides the energy we need. But as the sun sets, the body rests as part of a normal, natural cycle. But nighttime is the wrong time to eat. When we eat food, we stimulate ourselves, and in the process we are taking on more energy. You may not feel restful after eating in the evening. If that's the case, it's necessary to bring food consumption to an end at a considerably earlier time of the day.

If you feel very uncomfortable because of your hunger, it's permissible to have an easy-to-digest snack. In the beginning of dietary change, the feeling of discomfort could be being caused by your digestive system relieving itself of gas. Water is permissible as well: If you've made up your mind to stop eating at nighttime, keep plenty of good clean drinking water on hand.

If your energy is low and you want to change a particular vibration energetically in your body, you can add things like very ripe lemons to the water. But avoid cayenne or any sweetener—let the lemon do all the talking.

Perhaps you don't like citrus because you have an ulcer. If that's the case, then fix the ulcer first and then you can go back to citrus. You may believe that it's not possible to fix the ulcer, although you have no hard evidence to that effect. I'd advise you to have faith that the ulcer is curable. In the process you will instill confidence by thinking positive thoughts. Doing so will have an enormous positive impact on your chemistry.

If a large portion of your food consists of fresh foods that haven't been cooked and that exclude animal protein, you will begin a phenomenal process of healing. It will take time, and the amount of time is dependent on factors such as your existing chemistry and proper maintenance of your overall lifestyle.

As you become involved in the process of making such significant dietary changes, keep in mind a couple of things that have been covered earlier in this book. First of all, remember that this book is not a step-by-step instructional guide. It's an attempt to give a broad view of nutritional issues by way of actionable knowledge.

Secondly, always remember that in the course of making the dietary changes that this book section recommends, you must avoid processed junk foods like the plague. They will deter the process of healing that you are attempting to bring to fruition through positive dietary change.

And one thing pertaining to this topic bears repeating: It's clearly a mistake to have larger meals early in the evening. A social gathering with a big meal should happen in the morning rather than at night.

46. Food Cravings

Regarding miscellaneous cravings for unhealthy items, some of the following tips may be helpful. You might almost instinctively reach for a soda, a bottle of water, a beer, a smoothie, a piece of cake, another meal, a piece of kale, or a steak at any given time. Before you do so, you should ask yourself, "Is this really what I need right now?" Ask yourself that question frequently until it becomes an instinctive habit.

If you do that, you'll begin to develop greater self-awareness. Over time you'll find yourself answering "No" and then shifting to an activity or pursuit that will serve you better. As you do so, your thought processes will help you overcome your habitual craving(s).

If you ask your body if you're really hungry, your body may reply that you're thirsty or needing to be involved in a certain activity. So you might then get a drink of water or get involved in an activity that benefits you.

It's important to note that many people who are overweight don't take much, or any, pleasure from food. They eat for reasons other than hunger—primary deep-seated psychological reasons. (This was the case with my father.) If you identify yourself as the type of person who eats from such a compulsion, I urge you to employ the techniques pertaining to psychological issues that I discuss at some length in this book.

As you move along on your path toward weight control and good physical and mental health, your own consciousness will disclose to you certain things that no one else can. Quite a number of things have been helpful to me, and I include them as tips throughout this book.

I'd like to give you an example of one such thing that I do. On cool summer nights, I often go to a quiet place and look at the sky and am awed by the beautiful view. I count stars and try to figure out which of the bright objects I see are planets rather than stars. I imagine how it might be to get some distance from the earth and stare into space. I take long, deep breaths and think of how small I am compared to everything else out there.

This activity always helps me get away from my own compulsions, distractions, worries, and annoyances. When I do so, it's both a welcome break for me and a moment that I will treasure and come back to at some later point in time.

47. Sweet Tooth

There are a number of different kinds of overeaters. We all have different types of foods that we call comfort foods. We probably call them comfort foods for one of two reasons. One of the reasons is that when we eat such food it reminds us of something comforting: Something associated with love, or something that feels good other than (or in addition to) the taste of the food.

The other reason we can call that food comfort food is because our chemistry is so intoxicated by the substances in the food that we have tremendous cravings without it. The cravings can be very painful to the physical body because of agitation and discomfort in the mind. Usually when it's happening, we're not aware of the source.

A major transformation in the way that we look at food happens when we take the opportunity to become mindful when we have cravings for it. We should take a minute to think about what we're craving and try to connect it to an earlier source. For some people, it will require a lot of exploration to make such a connection.

I would venture to guess that the vast majority of the world's population experiences cravings for processed food. Because processed food can be intoxicating to the body, the body will store the toxic information to cause the craving. But the body can develop healthy cravings for nourishing foods in exactly the same way, provided that you train it to do so.

The body is a highly adaptable machine. It definitely adapts to what you feed it. That sets up the physical phenomena of craving for the things it adapts to, whether they be healthy substances or poisons. If you can become aware of your cravings and sit with each of those cravings a little longer each time, you'll get better at resisting them.

If you have cravings for sweets, as many do, and you eat candy to satisfy those cravings, you have what's called a "sweet tooth." Begging the question, where does your sweet tooth come from? Is it because you feel anxiety? Is it because the rush of processed sugar spikes you and gives you a momentary burst of excitement? Is it because you were wrongfully rewarded with candy by grownups when you were a child? These are important questions to ask and then write about. We all have to uncover such truth and expose it in order to work on overcoming these patterns.

For the most part in this book I leave out details about illnesses to fear. This is because I don't want to give people additional anxieties. Instead, I want to bring understanding of the causes and effects of everything that we put into our bodies.

If you have a sweet tooth, the next time a craving builds up make sure that you have a supply of fresh, delicious, ripe fruit available. Don't worry about the calories—you need to beat the craving first.

Make sure that you have apples, pears, strawberries, blueberries, and citrus fruit, depending on the time of day. I would recommend eating more caloric fruits earlier, when you're likely to be active. If your cravings are coming up at night, eat an apple. Or have a handful of blueberries.

You may be extremely concerned about the sugar if you have a blood sugar problem such as diabetes. If that is your situation, I recommend that you eat a celery stick with blueberries. When doing so, chew everything all the way until it's nothing. This can average the glycemic index of the food you're eating between the two different processes.

Please don't misunderstand what I'm saying to mean that you can or should eat 15 bananas when you have a sugar craving. It might be better to eat 15 bananas than to pig out on junk food, but overeating to such a degree is unwarranted.

I observed myself from time to time thinking and feeling that no matter how much food I ate I was left feeling hungry. Only two things prevented me from eating more: I physically could not handle putting anything more in my mouth, and I could not fit any more in my stomach.

When I thought about what the source of that insatiable hunger could have been, I realized that it connected back to a feeling of "being empty." It was a feeling that I was not connected to anything. It was a general feeling of being cut off from certain parts of my body. I felt as though I was floating in the universe alone with no purpose.

I still have that feeling from time to time, but very infrequently. I'm not sure exactly what causes the feeling, but when it surfaces I want sweet food first and then something heavy. The infrequent feeling occurs mostly at night as my mind is relaxing and my strength is lower.

Negative feelings then pulse in my chemistry. That leaves me in a state of confusion, because I am not hungry and I'm happy and feel physically great during such times. But there are still rare occasions during which I just can't feel satisfied. These are the times that I need to write, think, meditate, breathe, talk, sit still, or walk. And I need to keep things slow and mellow while doing so. I used to skydive to try and suppress these feelings; it never worked.

I may be the only person who feels the way I've just described and wants to eat when it happens—I'm not sure. Your particular motivations for eating too much, indulging in gluttony, eating junk food, drinking coffee in excess, or loading up on booze are likely different.

My suggestion is that you (as well as I) should look out for such moments and have a plan to involve yourself in a particular structured activity to overcome the craving. The more you do so, the more effective you will be at it, and you will have less likelihood of a relapse.

You may be saying to yourself, "F**k Antebi's nonsense. I don't have to give up desserts. I have to just change them to not include junk food. Every once in a while I can have crème brûlée, ice cream cake, chocolate cake from that gourmet restaurant, or movie concession candy."

If we allow ourselves to have that attitude, we will both do harm to our body chemistry and continue to have cravings, no matter how much "moderation" we exercise. In a sense, we are keeping our taste buds open, and they are anxiously looking forward to our next bad dietary decision.

When we surrender processed sugar from our diet, we are likely to experience a detox. Some find it easy and some don't. But it's advisable to eat plenty of fruit during this detoxing, provided that we're active enough to burn off some of the fruit sugar.

If you're a "need-a-dessert-once-and-while" kind of person, you may have to let this go if you want your new program to work for you. We must be willing to give up obvious junk food, even when it's served with a nice meal, at a nice place, and/or on a nice occasion. This is another highly critical adjustment to our lifestyles. Don't succumb to peer pressure, whatever kind of pressure it may be.

48. What the Heck Are We Really Craving?

Cravings are only a small part mental. The heavy toxic food dilemma is as follows: When you eat heavy, hard to process foods that are filled with all types of things that are negatively chemically addictive, you're going to crave them all day. You could eat a 3,000 calorie meal at 10 o'clock in the morning and then pile on a 1,500 calorie dessert. You'd think the amount of calories you consumed would make you good to go until the next day without having to eat another morsel of food.

But it doesn't work that way. You're going to find yourself picking at the turkey in the refrigerator, maybe throwing a little stuffing on it, and then suddenly you find yourself eating another meal. Eating to smother emotions sets up the phenomenon of craving.

But we're not actually craving more sustenance: We're craving the euphoric feeling of being full. Or we're eating to enjoy the activity because we're bored. Or the activity may be a distraction from sadness, depression, anger, anxiety, or another uncomfortable emotion.

It could also be that we want to feel something, anything. Putting food in the mouth conjures up a physical feeling. The textures, taste, and smell of food is an alteration of our present reality. We like that alteration so much that we bring ourselves into sickness and unhappiness.

Another likely thing that builds craving is eating "low conscious" foods that don't give us enough of the critical nutrients. This is a generalization, though, because deficiencies of nutrients vary widely from person to person. But such deficiencies are common. We do get carbohydrates, proteins and fat, and perhaps some vitamins and minerals in the unhealthy foods that we eat during cravings. But we get them at a significant cost, as these foods deplete our vitality and overall energy levels tremendously.

It is possible that your chemistry actually is saying, "I need more stuff." And in our lack of knowledge about what to reach for, we just reach for what's in the refrigerator and what tastes good. But when we do so, we're not getting the crucial nutrients that we need, especially the compounds that are in the great plant foods.

I've observed something in many, many people. The journey to a healthy diet, which likely will be linked to your personal happiness, entails discovering the things that you like within the boundaries that are set by someone who understands the chemistry of the body.

I've developed a good grasp of what my body needs, and I have a very good understanding of what is unhealthy for the human body. If you have cravings for something, that doesn't mean that you need it—it means that your body chemistry and your psychology want it. It doesn't mean that it's good for you.

•••

In the beginning of your dietary journey it's going to take time before you can trust your physical cravings. But over time they will change and become cravings for healthy food, provided that you devote yourself to healthy eating.

•••

An abstract concept that is not really science-based but that deserves consideration is as follows: When you eat things from the plant kingdom, they communicate with you—they communicate with your chemistry. People who don't believe in metaphysical things have difficulty understanding and/or accepting this. But I really don't think it's a metaphysical concept—I think it's basic science.

Consider the example of drinking a cup of coffee. The coffee is a plant, and that plant has a set of properties for its compounds. Those compounds will interact with your cells, setting off a chain reaction. There will be a communication that takes place from your cells to your brain, and from your brain back to your cells.

And as a result, your physiology will change. But there's another factor: Every single person reacts differently to those physiological changes that take place. Some people might hate the physical sensation that a cup of coffee will cause them to have, others will feel so stimulated that they'll feel euphoric. Most human beings will easily become addicted to anything that will make them feel good, let alone euphoric. That's why we're so attached to coffee.

As part of your healthy journey, it's important that if you've made up your mind to consume a certain thing, that you find the most optimal way to consume it. You should figure out a way to make it a very positive experience for your chemistry. You can then create the routine and habit around it and let your body's natural responses guide you. With boundaries, because at first your natural responses will be subtle, and you as a thinker will not be able to tap in and successfully control yourself.

49. How to See the Supermarket Experience

Go to the biggest supermarket that you know of with no intention of buying anything. Make sure that you're not hungry when you go. Walk through each and every aisle, look on every shelf, reach for all the different products that interest you, pick them up, and read the ingredients. Take phone pictures of desirable items that aren't processed foods. Also take pictures of aisles to avoid (e.g., the pastry aisle). Spend a lot of time in the produce aisle and take pictures of fresh and organic items. Imagine yourself to be a retail explorer trying to understand both trends in and the language of processed food.

Food companies copy each other. They use catchy names, attractive packaging, price points, and pretty colors. They use popular buzzwords such as "sugar free" or "low sugar," and include words such as "Paleo" on the packaging. And more often than not, what's in the package is utter garbage.

One of the things the supermarket journey exercise is intended to do is educate you about the forces working against you. Those forces are deceptive marketing techniques that food corporations often use, and they rely on the addictive behaviors, lack of knowledge, lack of discipline, and weaknesses of most consumers.

We're not deprived of good food choices at this time in the west. We have hundreds of plant-based, all natural, unprocessed choices available.

Next, make a list of produce types that you like. Those foods will be your staples; make sure that you purchase plenty of them when you shop. If you like vegetables, you are fortunate. Some suggested staples are avocados, apples, lemons, peaches, and plums. Have a bag of apples (organic only) handy at all times.

All produce should be organically seeded, grown, nurtured, harvested, and handled. "USDA Certified Organic" is the gold standard, indicating that good oversight and good natural hygienic practices took place during the growth and harvesting processes.

Any fruit that you eat the skin of must be organic, or else you're eating pesticides and wax, no matter how much you wash it.

50. Cravings and Emotional Food Attachments

If you eat things such as fried eggs and breakfast meats all your life, it's likely that you will have health problems when you get older. But **you can get your body to make the adjustment from eating processed food, meats, and foods high in fat and processed sugar to things like**

fresh fruit and vegetables. On a physical level, it doesn't take long for your body to get rid of those old foods and be really happy with the new ones. But psychologically it's somewhat harder.

We get accustomed to the feeling of the unhealthy foods as they hit our tongue and squish around in our mouth. It's like having an orgy, eating bacon and sausage and having your buttered toast to dip into the egg yolk. And what's more, when you eat that stuff your belly feels full. And a full belly usually communicates to the brain that everything is fine.

But over a reasonable length of time you can make an adjustment and get to the point that eating fruit will be just as exciting. We become desensitized when we are engaged in extremes; this applies to violence as well as to food. But we can adjust over time to let simple things stimulate us.

Slow and steady is boring for the western mind. Our TVs have to be 100 inches. The speakers have to be deafening. Our cars have to go faster, our credit cards have to have huge limits, our telephones have to do more and more things. And our diets have to be loaded with all kinds of extreme compounds that create extreme reactions.

That's why a nutrition book like this can even exist. Because a schmuck like me is trying to teach you how to detune your senses. I did so, and it took me a long time. It took me years to detox my eyeballs from craving Reese's peanut butter cups at the movies.

I ate that stuff to feel better as a compulsion. I wasn't hungry and I had other choices, but I had trained myself to reach for those cups and a giant soda. When I was younger, I couldn't have cared less about health, disease, illness, inflammation, or pain. I didn't feel any of that. But I set up my habits, my chemistry, and my cravings.

If I was not content and safe and feeling good in my life, I'd often be sitting in a cold movie theater watching some ridiculous fantasy movie with Arnold Schwarzenegger running around with his giant muscles blowing people up. I'd be eating a super-sized container of popcorn and the three delicious Reese's peanut butter cups that were creamy and loaded with sugar. My taste buds exploded.

My chemistry became sedated. I was drugged. When I watched those movies I was so drugged that I believed I was Arnold Schwarzenegger and that I could do those things that he was doing on the screen. I never went to a movie theater with a nectarine. "Nectarines are for pussies," I thought to myself.

Can you imagine movie theaters in the future that just served fresh fruit, clean drinking water, and maybe fresh juice? People would be sneaking in toxic food like kids sneaking drugs into a disco.

When you're reading this book, you're mostly on your own out there. If you're trying to figure out how to eat a healthy diet, a lot of weirdos like me out there can support you. But most of society will not give a shit. Everywhere in modern society we are surrounded by opportunities to succumb to our cravings or addictions in one way or another.

THE DIETARY CHANGE WORK

51. Eliminate Processed Food From Your Diet

At this point in this program, one thing should be perfectly clear: The number one most important thing that any person can do to improve their health and feel good about their diet is to eliminate all processed foods. There are different degrees to which foods and liquids are processed that determine how disruptive they will be to our chemistry. But we must rid ourselves of each and every food substance that disrupts our body chemistry.

Over the years, as I would talk to people in my retail business about diet, I found it really interesting how hard it was for people to connect with this simple concept: Eliminate processed food from your diet and you will feel better. First, the level of denial that people have about that subject is dumbfounding to me. I have encountered so many people who just don't want to believe in the simplicity of that premise.

In terms of weight loss, which is one of the foremost promises of this book, if you eliminate processed food and allow time for the adjustment to take place, then your entire eating pattern will change automatically. After a given point in time when your body has detoxed from the cravings, your chemistry will change. You will react to wholesome, pure, unadulterated foods completely differently than how you react to processed foods that have been tainted and perverted.

When foods are in their pure and natural state (for example, an apple or a piece of celery), because of the way they're designed and how your chemistry reacts to that design, you cannot overeat. This is an incredibly simple concept (as are most of the concepts that I write about). The problem is that the human mind is incredibly complex. So it's not necessarily easy for a person to let go of their behaviors.

This presents problems for the diet and health and wellness industries because the <u>truth</u> is not a scalable business. **Freshness and purity are the enemies of big profits!** Wholesome food spoils and rots easily, as it should. Good quality nutritious ingredients are more expensive than manufactured foods. Organic produce is more expensive than conventional produce. And even if wholesome food didn't spoil easily, and even if nutritious ingredients weren't expensive, a large population of humanity would still eat as if they were young children at a birthday party. This is disturbing for me to think about and try to communicate, and I take no pleasure in doing so. I'm just stating something that is an obvious truth—a truth that has caused so many problems in our collective health.

I dealt with that for years at JuicePress. People would look at the things that I wrote about health and nutrition and they would just say, "It's too hard. Can't you make it easier?" And I said to them, "No. I can help you with emotional support, but I can't bend the rules."

The secret or ultimate tip in your diet is to eliminate processed food first and foremost. And follow that guideline strictly. Do whatever it takes to get yourself to that state of existence. Don't settle for mediocrity. It's too common for people to believe that if they give up processed food "as much as they can handle" that they will feel better and that they will get things in order within their body.

That's not true. The way to approach giving up processed food is the same way a smoker has to approach quitting cigarettes. They have to become sick and tired of their unhealthy behavior, they have to reach a bottom, and then they have to muster up the courage and the strength to quit completely and quit for good.

Quitting things for good is only scary in the beginning because we have formed habits. Those habits somehow brought us comfort; emotional attachments were embedded into those habits. But we have to break our bad dietary habits. And then, each individual has to do something different that will help them connect to the foods that they eat.

What is food processing? Processed foods can either <u>make</u> your body chemically impure from its natural pristine starting point, <u>force</u> your chemistry to evolve in a way that it wasn't intended to, <u>prevent</u> your chemistry from evolving in the way it was designed to, or do all three. Scary stuff.

In a completely literal sense, processed food in its simplest form begins with food that you are chewing in your mouth. You are processing it just by masticating it. When you chew the food, it changes from its original state to a digestible state.

A blender processes food. A juice machine processes produce. But those processes don't alter the food in a way that transforms that food into something toxic or harmful to human chemistry. When you chew nuts, you're actually processing them into a pulverized matter that can be swallowed; if you didn't do so you'd choke on the nuts.

In the case of blending produce or juicing, this is minimal processing, so the result is not adulterating it or toxifying the juice.

The next form of processing food (that does cause the food to become adulterated) is when the food is cooked—specifically, when it's overcooked.

Manipulating temperature literally is alchemy. Cooking (manipulating temperature) changes food physically and alters it chemically.

It becomes a serious issue when you are unintentionally causing the food to become something that isn't compatible with human chemistry. Anything that isn't compatible with your physical chemistry is essentially something that is toxic, so your body then has to work hard to remove it.

There are different ways to create toxic food. One way is to cook something at a very high temperature for a long time. Doing so reduces it to its basic elemental form in which the compounds become concentrated and more difficult for the body to break down.

This is especially the case with refined sugar (processed and heated sugar). It's a similar situation with salt. When it's natural (from the ocean or from a salt mine), it's a mineral that is essential to body chemistry. But when it's heated, the chemistry of the salt compound changes, making it adulterated.

Fats can be extracted from a number of plants and concentrated. But elements can be added to them that make them completely incompatible with the body's chemistry.

52. Toxic Food Processing

The next level of processed food (primarily food that contains additives) consists of foods that have been changed from their original, easily digestible forms. Sometimes they're changed into forms that make them more difficult to digest.

Become very mindful about what processed foods are. If you look on the back of a food package to see the ingredients, if you don't see just fruits and vegetables, a small amount of spices, and perhaps an all-natural sweetener such as maple syrup, keep looking. If you then see many items that look like the names of pharmaceutical medicines, it's probably processed food.

Most boxes that I've seen that had pictures of animal figures or drawings of fruits and vegetables usually contained very heavily processed foods. Such artwork is often a deceptive advertising ploy.

There are quite a number of artificial chemicals that are legally used and permitted by the governmental agencies in different countries that regulate commercially produced foods in different countries. In the United States, that agency is the Food and Drug Administration. Their regulatory system is so unbelievably corrupt that that subject alone could comprise five lengthy books. But for the moment I'm going to leave the FDA alone and just blame the food product manufacturers for their corrupt ways.

The processed food industry is not much different than the cigarette industry. They manipulate foods to make consumers addicted to their products. Subsequently, people will buy many of those products, and the industry players will have wonderful profits every quarter. The food scientists that serve these companies are well aware of the nasty and toxic side effects that these compounds have on human chemistry, and they apparently don't care.

The short list of nasty processed foods begins with anything that is refined down to the point where there's nothing left but the desired compound, such as is the case with sugar. Sugar is naturally occurring in almost every plant that we eat. With an extraction and heat process followed by refinement and then more heat, those naturally occurring sugars can be turned into something mind-blowingly sweet.

Processed sugar is a great offender, but there are many, many other great offenders. Think of the grapes in the wine you drink and ask yourself, "Does processed food such as the grapes in my wine include anything that's been sprayed 100 times with varieties of pesticides?" The answer to that is absolutely yes. If you have a hard time believing that, then I'll come to your house with an eyedropper and I'll put a drop of that pesticide on your fingertips and say, "Please put that on your tongue: It's the pesticides they are spraying on your grapes." There's no way that you would be interested in tasting the pesticide. But for some reason we forget that our produce is doused in pesticides. Certainly you could wash off some of it, but not the pesticides that leach into the soil and leach into the fibers of the produce.

Now, consider the livestock industry. Ask yourself what is in the beef that you are eating. Are there traces of antibiotics that they fed the animal throughout its life to prevent it from illness and spreading disease? Are there growth inducing hormones that are synthetically pumped into the animal's feed?

Look at the back side of all the products that are in the best supermarkets. The most important thing about anything that you eat is its ingredients. They will be listed in the smallest print on the box. It's much more important to the company to get their logo out there and any marketing messages deployed to win you over.

That must shift. The most important thing that should be on the front side of a box of food is the name of the company, their highest values, and every ingredient in a 19-point font. If any ingredient is synthetically manufactured or refined and processed there should be an asterisk next to the ingredient. And the asterisk should refer to a statement at the bottom of the box or bag saying that the product will cause you harm in the long run.

One day in the future, the Food and Drug Administration will require foods to be packaged in this way. But not today. Today you have to be a well-informed consumer. You have to vote with your dollars. If enough people stay away from the garbage that's put into the supermarkets, those companies will have to change their ways. On the website *www.goodsugar.life*, I have posted articles that I will leave up there for the next 100 years that have a list of everything that's out there that's processed and not good for your health. The list is long.

Avoid all pasteurized dairy purchased in supermarkets. If you're going to consume dairy, which I strongly advise against you doing, make sure that it comes from an animal about the same size as yourself that you milk yourself.

If you're going to eat the flesh of an animal, make sure you are clear on where it was raised and what food it ate for its entire life (even the last few weeks before its death). There's a scam that's currently used in the industry. Packages can claim that the beef is grass fed, but they can still feed the animals corn in the last two or three months of their lives. By doing this the producers can both save money and fatten their animals considerably before they are killed.

Do you really want to eat corn? If you are eating an animal that's fed corn, you're eating corn indirectly. Not that there's anything wrong with corn, but why not just eat corn in its raw form and let the other animal live?

There are a great many food products and seasonings you need to stay away from for the sake of your health, including white sugar, granulated sugar, powdered sugar, corn syrup, maltodextrin, and soy products.

THE goodsugar DIET™

Below is a short list of the most dangerous food additives, colorings, and preservatives used in today's processed foods:

- ▶ Sodium nitrate: This is added to foods such as processed meat products in order to stop bacterial growth. It's been linked to cancer in humans and is considered one of the most unhealthy of all food additives.
- ▶ Recombinant Bovine Growth Hormone (rBGH): This is a genetically modified chemical that causes growth and milk production in cows and is believed to cause different types of cancer.
- ▶ Sodium benzoate: This is used in carbonated beverages, salad dressings, and other products as a preservative. It's known to cause cancer and is suspected to damage DNA as well.
- ▶ Carnauba wax: This product, which can cause tumors and cancer, is used as a glaze in various foods and is contained in chewing gums as well.
- ▶ Orange B: This product is toxic to the liver and bile duct. It's a dye commonly used in sausage casings and hot dogs.
- ▶ Carrageenan: This is widely used in prepared foods as a thickening agent and a stabilizer, and it can cause both cancer and ulcers.
- ▶ BHA/BHT: This extends shelf life in foods by serving as a fat preservative. It has been shown to be a factor in the growth of cancerous tumors.
- ▶ Yellow #6: This carcinogenic additive is believed to cause kidney tumors. It's widely used in beverages, baked goods, and sausage.

- Aluminum: It can cause cancer when it is used in packaged foods as a preservative.
- Monosodium glutamate (MSG): This is used to enhance flavor in many products. It causes many people to have headaches. Studies have also linked it to seizures, heart problems and nerve damage.
- Paraben: This is a preservative used to stop yeast formation and mold. It disrupts hormones in the body and may be linked to breast cancer.
- Yellow #5: This dye is commonly used in baked goods, candy, and desserts, and studies suggest that kidney tumors are caused by it.
- Sulfites: They are widely used to enhance the freshness of prepared foods. The ingredient causes many individuals who are sensitive to it to have difficulties in breathing.
- Brown HT: This additive, which can cause cancer, asthma, and child hyperactivity, is found in a wide variety of packaged foods.
- Red #40: This is very commonly used as a food coloring in products. It is made from petroleum (as are many food dyes) and it's linked to both child hyperactivity and cancer. A number of European countries have banned its use.
- Propyl gallate: This is added to products that contain fat and is linked to cancer.
- Olestra: This is used widely in snack foods instead of natural fat. It is bad for the heart and causes many people to have digestive problems.

- Red #3: This is commonly used in bakery goods, pie fillings, and ice cream. It can cause thyroid cancer and nerve damage.
- Chlorine dioxide: This product, which is used to bleach flour, causes tumors as well as child hyperactivity.

Next is a short list of some of the most dangerous processed foods that are now on the market:

- Sodas: in addition to having no nutritional value and having an outrageous amount of sugar, they use high-fructose corn syrup, which is damaging to the liver. Many diet sodas contain carcinogenic sweeteners that perpetuate cravings for real sugar as well.
- White bread: contains a great deal of processed sugar for added flavor, is stripped of all nutritional value, and uses chemicals such as benzoyl peroxide that can cause headaches, nausea, and dna damage.
- Hot dogs and processed meats: these have sodium nitrate and other dangerous compounds in them and are linked to stomach and bowel cancers as well as high blood pressure and heart disease.
- Cookies and cakes: most of these products can contain up to 80 ingredients, most of which are harmful additives such as preservatives and artificial coloring. Most also contain partially hydrogenated oils with trans fats, which are associated with diabetes, coronary heart disease, and alzheimer's.

- Quick noodle soups: one package can contain up to 2,000 milligrams of sodium, greatly exceeding the american heart association's recommended daily limit of 1,500 milligrams per day. This puts frequent users at risk of high blood pressure or a stroke
- Microwave popcorn: one serving can contain 270 milligrams of sodium and 8 grams of fat; the american heart association recommends a maximum of 11 to 13 grams of saturated fat per day. The microwaveable bags contain chemicals such as perfluoroalkyls, linked to poor semen quality and impaired kidney function.
- Frozen dinners: they have outrageously high contents of sugar, fat, and sodium, which can raise blood pressure and lead to heart and weight problems. The most popular of these products contain between 1,100 to 1,300 milligrams of sodium.
- Fast food iced tea: it contains propylene glycol alginate, which is also used in de-icer and antifreeze automotive products. It can cause neurotoxic and cardiovascular problems.
- Candy: besides excess processed sugar, candy contains many very toxic and carcinogenic chemicals used for artificial coloring and other purposes; they include yellow number 5 and yellow number 6, linked to attention deficit disorder in children.
- Sugary cereal: in addition to incredibly high sugar content, it contains chemicals such as butylated hydroxytoluene (BHT) and that are believed to be carcinogenic. (Those ingredients are banned in many European countries.)

- Energy drinks: they contain excessive amounts of sucrose, glucose, and caffeine, as well as toxic artificial sweeteners. One study found that they are more corrosive to teeth than sodas.
- Ice cream: most varieties contain artificial coloring, soybean oil, and titanium dioxide (a chemical used in sunblock), as well as a tremendous amount of sugar.
- Breakfast biscuits: these are very high in trans fats that can cause heart disease. Some products that are labeled as having 0 grams of trans fats contain hydrogenated soybean oil, meaning that traces of fat actually are in the products.
- Macaroni and cheese: it contains yellow number 5 and yellow number 6 and coal tar (which is used to seal floors and kill bugs in shampoo). Those additives can cause adhd and allergies, and they are suspected to be linked to cancer as well.
- Margarine: although it's considered by some to be a better choice than butter, it contains trans fats that lowers good cholesterol levels and is linked to heart disease. It is high in omega-6 fatty acids that cause a chemical imbalance between omega-3 and omega-6 acids, potentially causing bodily inflammation. Dangerous chemicals are used in its production as well.
- Bacon: this is probably the worst of the processed meats available. It tastes delicious primarily because it's extremely high in saturated fats (that cause obesity and heart disease). The preservatives that are used, including nitrates, are considered to be carcinogenic.

- ▶ Instant ramen: although it's a popular product among those on tight budgets, it's incredibly unhealthy and has almost no nutritional value. A typical portion of it has about 1,500 milligrams of sodium and 14 grams of fat, and it also contains additives such as msg (monosodium glutamate).
- ▶ Coffee creamer: it's loaded with trans fats and the chemical whitening product called titanium dioxide, which may cause liver and tissue damage. The trans fats in the hydrogenated oil used can cause diminished memory in adults.
- ▶ Baked goods: these use potassium bromide, also known as bromated flour, to speed up cooking processes. It's found in wraps, bagel chips, and commercial bread crumbs. The dangerous chemical used is believed to cause cell deterioration and kidney failure, and it has been banned in canada and europe.
- ▶ Jam and jelly: besides being loaded with sugar, they contain high quantities of pectin. Pectin is toxic because it attaches to good, healthy antioxidants including lycopene, beta-carotene and others, causing them to be eliminated from your system before they can provide health benefits to your body.
- ▶ Chewing gum: although it's not a food as such, it contains butylated hydroxyanisole (bha) which is released into your body when you chew the product. Bha has been linked to impairment of blood clotting and to tumor growth as well. BHA has been banned from use in food products in many European countries and Japan.

53. Diet Plan Considerations

I've become aware of an unusual contradiction in the weight loss paradigm. The contradiction lies within the false notion that permanent weight loss can be achieved by manipulating your calories in and your calories out. Sadly, this is more or less the standard model for most modern diets.

Fad diets offer the allure of rapid weight loss. Few people are aware of the long-term mental and physical consequences of this path to weight loss. It's promised that weight loss can be achieved through taking pills, eating lots of fat and/or protein, eliminating all carbohydrates, and other measures. But such diets are essentially "chemistry cheats."

If you're overweight by any amount and create a biologically compatible human diet for yourself, your necessity to count calories will be reduced dramatically. You could likely stay on the same calorie count that you had before with junk food and other unhealthy products.

Just by changing the type of food that you're eating, from bad to good, you will lose weight. You will feel much better. Physically you will become healthier from the inside out. It will likely take longer than the length of time that a popular fad diet might suggest, but you will lose the weight and you will keep it off. And isn't that the goal, to live a healthier life for a longer amount of time? I've seen this happen literally thousands of times.

But there are a couple of catches to this type of diet plan. One is that you need to stay with it—you cannot relapse. And two, you will need to do a lot of "work." What I mean by "work" is the intellectual and emotional deep dive into your current habits and behaviors. You have the strength within yourself to do this work.

Some people might not be prepared to break food addictions "cold turkey." They may have to work their way into better patterns gradually. Such people will benefit from this book, because this book isn't about a quick fix for overnight weight loss.

This is a marathon, not a sprint. This book is about introducing new habits, repeating them, absorbing them, and folding them into your life. Two critical aspects needed to set yourself up for success with this plan are eating well and having peace of mind. Peace of mind is crucial to control your negative impulses for the long term.

If you need to drop weight quickly, you will need to not only clean up your diet immediately but also count calories. You will need to go into a calorie deficit to shed the pounds.

Such fast paced weight loss will create a problem, though. Mostly because it is psychologically unsound to lose weight too fast for your psyche to handle. **Your mind will want the old calories and the old body back. The reason is that the mind creates the body the way it has for good reason: Your psychological survival.**

The mind has to make the adjustment to a new body slowly. If not, it will work hard to get back to what it knows, forcing you to eat at a higher volume. This is because it wants to return to a sense of normal, even if that "normal" is unhealthy and/or uncomfortable in the long run.

It's possible that you'll gain the weight back and feel demoralized if that happens. Subsequently you may go into a tailspin of sorts. You may become anxious and revert to eating unhealthy comfort foods.

•••

If you follow this program, then you can avoid all of this. If you mess up, I advise you to be compassionate to yourself and try again. This method works, and it works for the long haul.

•••

Give yourself time, but set realistic goals and expectations regarding your weight loss. The very first thing you should do is educate yourself on what you should eat and what you should avoid eating. You can find quite a bit of detailed information regarding that in sections 54 through 88 in this book.

54. Food Disorder Syndromes

I have studied the multiple types of food disorders, with their origins dating back thousands of years—from the advent of large-scale agriculture, the transport and distribution of grains, and the reliance on livestock. These disorders fall into the following categories:

- ▶ Misinterpretation of what is food for humans.
- ▶ Dependency on stimulation for mood adjustments.
- ▶ Eating processed foods.
- ▶ Eating while angry and distracted.
- ▶ Pleasure eating versus eating to satiate hunger.
- ▶ Laziness to go after food from nature ("Let the king do it—I will just pay taxes."): "Grab and go eating" for the sake of convenience.

- ▶ Being disconnected from food while eating it (for example, so-called "zombie eating" while staring at a computer or TV screen).
- ▶ Being cogs in the wheel of large-scale agriculture with the massive food distribution industry, rather than individuals in a society being involved with food gathering. (Today food gathering is disconnected from the sounds and smells of nature. We connect with foods in supermarkets. Even when we purchase beautiful food, we can't connect with it as if we were living in nature.)
- ▶ The reliance on livestock for food sources, transferring an entire paradigm of cruelty from farm to table: Cruelty therefore creates and permeates the subtle undertones that weave the fabric of our societies.
- ▶ Compulsive eating, meaning eating when we do not want to out of a compulsion that usually originates from anxiety.
- ▶ Inability to eat mindfully.
- ▶ Eating too much (overeating).
- ▶ Eating too little (undereating).
- ▶ Not eating with gratitude for having food: Inability to eat gratefully.
- ▶ Being disconnected from the forces that foods have on our bodies.
- ▶ Eating late at night (doing so causes indigestion and other chemistry problems).

Most of the underlying concepts related to eating disorders are psychological in nature. This being the case, it's very important to understand the psychology behind our unhealthy eating practices and how to overcome those barriers to health and wellness.

To achieve lifelong changes with respect to our eating, we must learn to reorganize our thinking around all of the toxic habits we have created with respect to food. Once we do so, we become ready to eliminate them.

55. Addictive Food Types

Many food types are addictive, in the sense that when they're ingested they cause cravings for it to a degree beyond what the body requires for nutrition. Two in particular are processed sugar and concentrated protein.

Processed sugar is extremely addictive. This type of sugar is different from sugars that naturally occur in fruits and starchy vegetables. Natural sugar is not concentrated, and it relates to your chemistry in a way that makes your body feel satisfied. You may crave fruit, but the craving will feel natural. The craving for processed sugar can feel extremely overwhelming.

• •

When it is in a concentrated form, protein is addictive as well. The body needs protein, but not a great deal of it. In flesh foods, protein is concentrated to a degree that is beyond what is needed by the body. Plant foods are a preferable source of protein.

• •

Elimination of most processed food from your diet should be a top priority for you. In place of these foods, you must consume healthy food products. It will require some study and effort on your part to determine what some of those products should be. But doing so will pay off tremendously in the long run.

56. Supermarket Food Issues

If you try walking through the supermarket and staring at ingredients, you will become amazed at how little is offered other than produce in the way of clean, unadulterated food.

It's not that companies don't want to provide that type of food: It's that it's costly for them to do so. Fresh foods spoil easily, pure foods aren't that popular, and they take up prime real estate in refrigerators and freezers in supermarkets. Freshness is the greatest enemy of profits because there is more waste. Supermarkets like shelf-stable foods, and so do their clients.

I use two terms in particular describing these situations. I often refer to highly processed foods as "perverted" foods. And I often refer to fresh foods as "prude" foods. Prude foods are really shy. They don't show up very often in your supermarket, and sometimes they're hard to find. All the foods in the produce section that are organic are very prude.

Foods that are genetically modified have been perverted in some way. They've been corrupted. And we may not know all of the negative effects that will occur later if we eat them. But they are not the way they would have been in the Garden of Eden or even in your neighborhood farm stand. They are not completely natural.

I'm trying to give you concepts that you can implement to improve your lifestyle. I'm telling you to go to the supermarket and figure out what products you should stay away from.

If you walk through the meat, poultry and fish sections of your local supermarket, the products might be displayed beautifully. But you'd know nothing about the unhealthy processes behind their preparation. Things are added to, subtracted from, and altered in such a way that eating them will make you and your children sick.

Supermarkets and retail grocery stores of all sizes throughout the world have proverbial poison berry bushes—rancid, foul sources of toxic material—in every aisle. We arrived at this problem slowly but surely because of the following reasons: (1) people succumb easily to temptation; (2) food corporations seized the opportunity created by this vulnerability; and (3) our addiction to bad food runs incredibly deep in our cultures. As long as there is a multi-trillion dollar industry enabling us, humanity will likely be unable to get control over its problems with food, diet-related illness, and diet-related death.

Get out of that loop. It sucks. You are beautiful. You deserve happiness. You deserve to have a pristine and pure body. Make a choice to stop eating toxic food. Read the next paragraph—digest its words:

<u>Fruits, vegetables, nuts, sprouts and seeds are the optimal fuel for the human body</u>. The more active one is, the more calories one needs to consume. Plants can and do provide more than adequate quantities of all of the nutrients needed, including protein. If the nutrient that you think you need is not available in the plant kingdom, your body does not need it. That includes any substance that becomes a hot trend in the health industry, from collagen to vitamin k1. If there is no plant source of it, human chemistry does not need it.

Without question, processed foods are far more detrimental to our chemistry than any other dietary mistake. This is the thing we need to concentrate most of our effort on in order to have a clean diet—the elimination of all processed foods. (Alcohol, including wine, is a form of processed food.)

Changing a lifetime of eating processed food is not something that I would expect anyone to achieve overnight, with the exception of if one were sick and their life depended on a radical and immediate dietary shift. In such a case I'd recommend the following under no uncertain terms: Eliminate all processed foods, alcohol, and animal protein, and follow the rest of the concepts of this book precisely.

For others with generally good health who are making changes to their diet, elimination of processed food will likely be a gradual, step-by-step process. This should be done by first eliminating the processed foods that are the most dangerous.

In my opinion, the most dangerous processed foods are candies, cakes, white flour, refined processed sugars, foods containing preservatives, foods grown using pesticides, soda, beer, energy drinks, fast foods, fried foods, and many of the snacks that are found at 24-hour convenience stores. Most of these foods are made with complete and utter disregard for health and are mostly targeted towards children and busy, stressed-out adults.

All of these items cause the slow or fast destruction of what should be a pristine and pure body chemistry. They have no redeeming value whatsoever, except that they can provide you with some calories, energy, and flavor explosions in the mouth.

Processed bread, processed meats, and fried foods — these are all a scourge to mankind. These types of foods have waged a somewhat silent war on humanity. They are so pervasive now that it's not even considered questionable to eat them.

Particularly in Caribbean countries and poor nations in the world, it's shocking to see how retail businesses thrive on selling their garbage for the consumption of human beings. I find it hard to believe that doing so is legal. In my opinion, the most dangerous of the processed foods are weapons of mass destruction. They qualify as slow-killing chemical weapons, and they are targeted primarily toward youth and toward the ill-informed.

57. Nutrition: An Overview

Our body is made up of atoms and molecules, and in the process of living you use them up. The purpose of eating food is to replace them.

•••

When we eat food we are looking to obtain nutrients, because nutrients are beneficial to the body. The nutrients that your body needs a lot of cannot be created by a body on its own. There are two classifications of nutrients: macronutrients and micronutrients.

•••

Macronutrients are carbohydrates, proteins, and fat. Micronutrients are substances that the body produces on its own in small amounts and gets more of from the food that you eat and supplements you take.

Food can have other beneficial compounds. They include phytochemicals, antioxidants, and flavonoids. Along with macronutrients and micronutrients, they help the body perform its mechanical processes.

The body of a human being is a carbohydrate-burning machine; our entire anatomy, chemistry and physiology are set up to primarily use carbohydrates for functionality.

The carbohydrates that we were intended to eat come from fruits and vegetables. These are our primary source of energy. The energy that is contained in the plant-based foods is energy that came directly from the sun: The plant was able to convert the sun's energy into its own tissue.

The energy from the sun is the first source of energy for all living creatures on this planet. Plants are the only living creatures that can convert the energy of the sun into energy that it can use to conduct its mechanical functions.

58. What Is Food?

This subsection title may seem to be a no-brainer, but it really isn't. There is a great deal of misinformation and even flat out deception presented about this topic. To understand the proper steps to take to improve diet and related lifestyle choices, most people need to be retaught what food is in the first place. We need strong signals—similar to stop signs and green lights, metaphorically—to tell us what to do and what to eat or avoid eating.

Food is fuel (a source of energy) for an organism. The requirement for a substance to be given the elevated status of being called food, it must meet the following standards:

- ► Originate naturally from earth (rather than being a synthetic product from a laboratory),
- ► Provide energy or compounds (elements) that the body can use to repair itself,
- ► Not be toxic to the body,
- ► Be compatible with a human's digestive organs and our unique chemistry.

The first primary nutrient is air—the air that we breathe actually has nutritional value. In breathing through the nose and mouth, we absorb the most fundamental basic compound for our life. We force it into the lungs, and the lungs digest it and the nutrients in it. The air subsequently goes into the bloodstream so that we live.

The next fundamental element we consume is water—something that we need to be extremely grateful for. Each and every day of our lives we should take a moment to look at water and see it as some kind of blessing. (This is essential for activating the power of water in your body; whether or not you even believe that, practice being grateful for water. Over time those positive words and thoughts about it will kick in.)

59. Plant-Based: The Optimal Diet for Humans

People are eager to start on the path to a healthy diet. But what I learned through watching people at Juice Press is that they get tripped up because of erroneous informational roadblocks. The content in this book should be the final word on every subject related to food and should enable you to stop worrying.

We changed millions of peoples' lives reminding them to leave out processed foods and adopt a plant-based diet. This is what I recommend for you.

At this point, I ask you to not dismiss my recommendations or throw this book away. You work against yourself if you discard anything that advocates positive change. In my understanding and experience, a clean and highly pure diet might be difficult to put into practice, but it is something well worth the effort, and the results will blow your mind.

So, you may ask, what am I supposed to eat? I am not willing to offer meal-to-meal instructions. One thing that you will need to do is work hard on your own and research concepts regarding proper dietary choices. But I will give you quite a few suggestions that you'll find to be helpful.

• •

In order to reach health and weight goals, I recommend eating at least one large leafy green salad with any mixture of vegetables, preferably raw, every day of your life (for the rest of life, no days off). In addition to that, have at least one fruit every day. For best results, change up the fruit in order to get a variety of nutrients into your diet.

• •

Change-ups are good. You do not need to add flesh foods for protein to every salad (or any salad, for that matter). If you want a protein boost, add vegetables high in protein such as broccoli. You must make certain that you get enough total calories for your daily needs to ensure that you're getting your necessary nutrients.

As I see it, one of the problems with traditional diet programs is that they offer specific products and meal plans to customers in such a way that the consumers are not required to become well-versed in the sciences (or lack of them), issues of practicality, and nutritional benefits or liabilities behind them. Essentially, such diets enable us to be "unmindful."

Ultimate healing and recovery entails being mindful of your actions, especially around eating. This requires a great deal of thinking about food. It requires stopping the angry, sometimes childlike behavior of remaining disconnected from your food—disconnected from its rhythms and the intense vibrations that are an integral part of what food is and does.

•••

You have to engage in this process of weight reset and control. You have to learn. You have to research. You have to stop letting other people do those things for you. Only then can you heal your dysfunctional relationship with food and enjoy it in the way that it is intended and designed for you.

•••

60. Fear of Not Getting Enough Protein in Your Diet

You do not need any animal flesh to survive. You can consume some animal flesh if you need to—that is your choice. Every nutrient that the human body needs is available from the plant kingdom. Always has been and always will be. One of the most common things that I hear from people who want to start reducing their intake of animal proteins is that they're fearful of not getting enough protein.

I'll begin by saying that a person who is not an expert in food doesn't even really know what protein is. They know that it's a source of energy but they have no idea how it works, what the prime molecular drivers are, and how much the body really needs at any given stage of life.

A newborn needs a tremendous amount of protein in their diet, and that's why mother's milk is so rich in protein. A child's basic physical needs are to maintain the rapid growth and development of the organs, the bones, and the muscles. The amount of protein that we need in childhood is significantly larger than what is needed in the later years post childhood. As our physical growth plateaus, our protein needs decrease. As we age, protein, if taken in excess, it will become a burden on our body chemistry. It will intoxicate us. We can only process as much protein as we can use. This is based on your activity levels, your overall size, and the stage of development you are at in your life.

As I've said before in many of my writings, people mistake the craving for protein for the actual need for protein. The two are different.

Protein, like carbohydrates, is a substance that our body will call for based on how much of it the body is used to. If you reduce your protein intake, your chemistry will crave the amount it was used to prior to your dietary changes.

All the great masters of food agree that too much protein is a problem in the western diet, not a solution. In the context of a young guy in the gym lifting ridiculous amounts of weight trying to grow to an enormous size, protein is his solution. But it will be a consequence to his athleticism and his overall health somewhere down the line caused by the problems that too much protein creates in anyone's body chemistry.

If you choose to use an animal protein as a source of calories, no one should judge you. You need to do what you feel is best, but I remind you (over and over again), you truly don't need animal protein to thrive.

In any case, it's your journey. Remember that the best source of protein comes from the plant kingdom. This bears repeating! We need to hear it over and over again and apply it to our lives.

The flesh of an animal does not contain any special substance that does not exist in the plant kingdom as well. If the nutrient substance you are seeking does not exist in the plant kingdom, your body does not need it.

This is a raging debate in nutrition circles. But it's been my experience that the people who hold onto the animal protein paradigm are people who simply do not want to surrender flesh foods from their own diets. So flesh eating is what they teach.

I don't like to be judgmental, but I firmly believe this is the case. There is a great deal of scientific evidence to support this position.

In conclusion to this protein-focused section, if you are getting enough calories from a broad spectrum of foods, preferably plant-based foods, you'll be getting enough total nutrients, including protein, fat, carbohydrates, vitamins, and minerals. Deficiencies in any of those nutrients can be linked to other causes.

The following are good plant-based sources of protein:

- ▶ Plant-based, USDA protein powders made from any one of these or combinations of them: Hemp, pea, pumpkin, brown rice, or other nutrient-rich plants. (There are many different companies making protein powders. Read the ingredients and avoid ones that are made with stevia and other processed ingredients.)

▶	Broccoli	▶	Black beans
▶	Tempeh	▶	Hemp seeds
▶	Quinoa	▶	Lentils
▶	Collards	▶	Nut milks
▶	Chia seed	▶	Peas
▶	Spinach	▶	Kale
▶	Sprouts	▶	Corn
▶	Mushrooms	▶	Brussels Sprouts
▶	Artichoke	▶	Asparagus
▶	Edamame	▶	Arugula

61. Change Your Dietary Perspective

Hopefully by now you realize that effective eating requires more than just changing the particular products that you consume. Effective eating requires soul searching, lifestyle changes, deep introspection, and other actions that are difficult at first, but extremely beneficial in the long run.

In my weight loss program, I want to change our worlds around. I don't want you to think of loss—I want you to think about finding your body. The approach has to be layered, integrated and devoid of concepts such as counting calories and attempting to change the shape of our body to fit into a bikini or a tuxedo. Hopefully, this far into my writings, you've learned that actions like that are not sustainable.

In a future book I intend to give you a structured program that you can follow. Right now, though, it's necessary to focus on philosophy and patterns of thinking.

•••

Our eating patterns should be designed around our hunger and our bodies calling for sustenance to keep their functions going. And to a degree, those things depend on our individual activity levels and personality structures.

•••

We must consider our diet in the year 2020 and not eat in ways that will lead to sickness. In our diets, we must consider how much stimulation we think we require. And individuals must design for themselves programs that accommodate their social needs. Yet eating should not be unduly influenced by social desires at the expense of health, including meals that we would ordinarily have with our families.

If you have preconceived notions that your religious scriptures tell you to eat until you are stuffed, then you are misinterpreting the teachings. The body is a temple that must be respected. Eating is actually a high sacrament—and this will be something that you will feel as you begin to reclaim your body.

In my program, it's necessary to say kind things directly to our bodies while looking at them—because these words have a powerful effect, whether you believe so or not. We've said mean things in our heads to our bodies for too long. Part of the healing process is to change those unkind words into beautiful songs. We will cover positive thinking and gratitude in upcoming sections of this book.

62. Food Is Fuel, Not Medicine

Now, solid food, the third primary nutrient after air and water, needs to be considered. Solid foods should be regarded as fuel for our bodies, which are incredibly complex and marvelous machines. I like to think of our prime sources of fuel (food) using terms that are easier to relate to:

- Carbohydrate: New name; Prime Fuel/Source of Energy #1.
- Protein: New name; Cell Rebuilder, Fuel Source #2.
- Fat: New name; Insulator/Protector of the Cellular World, Fuel Source #3.

Vitamins and minerals are also nutrients, but they provide little to no energy. They provide the compounds that connect processes vital to life. The vitamins and minerals are present in our fuels 1, 2, and 3. If we select foods correctly, they provide ample energy while being accompanied by vitamins and minerals.

One of the most incredible things about our bodies is the healing capabilities that they possess. The metaphor of man-made machines is quite applicable: It can be helpful to think of our bodies as the remarkable machines that they are, and the foods we eat as replacement parts that the body needs for repair and recovery.

But it's necessary to keep in mind that the compounds from food can do nothing in and of themselves. Healing occurs through the interaction of our bodies with the foods that we eat. And it's necessary to have both a clean, nutritious diet and a sound mind. You must think of good things continually and direct your attention to bodily wellness to facilitate the miraculous healing processes that your body engages in. Food is not medicine and medicine is not food. Your body is self-healing when you eliminate the wrong food and include the right food. Your body functions are the medicine if the components needed are present. When the body's pathway to recovery is blocked, medicine may be the intervention that is needed. Medicine or healing compounds are not necessarily edible foods—they may be medicinal only.

63. What Is Not Food?

Any substance that disrupts the body's natural chemistry is not really food. It may have calories and some other nutrients, but it's not food. It's junk food. A substance that enhances the body's natural chemistry is technically food. Many edible products manufactured today do not qualify as food. Some foods are physically and chemically processed to the degree that they have little or no nutritional value, and they are often very harmful to a person's health.

This realization is many of several big realignments that we need to come to. Processed foods may have some nutrients, but they are still not food because they intoxicate the body. And very often, over time, eating processed foods leads to sickness. Interestingly, while all of humanity struggles to find the best sources of fuel for our machines and technologies (e.g., fossil fuels, wind power, solar power, nuclear power), we are also struggling to find the cleanest fuel sources for our bodies.

This isn't coincidental—the two problems are linked. It's a breakthrough when we understand the consciousness required to meet the needs for energy without destroying the organism—whether it be energy for cities or energy for the individual organisms that live in them.

I can offer you tools to establish what should NOT be in your diet, and then the diet that suits your body best will fall into place.

There are some places that I avoid like the plague. There is not a single item that I would consider "food" at that really famous donut franchise, for example.

There are very few places that I shop for food. And sometimes even when I go into those places I get annoyed, because I look at all the deception that health food stores still practice: Labels that try to make processed food seem healthy or natural with branding and imagery and fake titles like "Paleo" to distract from the highly processed ingredients inside.

64. Understand Nutritional Needs and Principles: Misconceptions Regarding Nutrition

A while back, I created a survey and asked 100 Juice Press customers (from as wide an age range and demographic as possible from this group) what they thought the most important nutrient for humans is.

- ▶ Seventy-five percent (70%) said they believed that protein was the most important nutrient.

- ▶ Twenty percent (20%) stated carbohydrates (most just stated fruits and vegetables, not being aware that they are primarily carbohydrates).

- ▶ Five percent (5%) stated a number of outrageously incorrect things: e.g., fat, bread (which isn't a nutrient but a food group containing carbohydrates), vitamin C, anything with calcium, and milk (which isn't a nutrient but a food category).

- ▶ Five percent (5%) couldn't care less and just wanted a free juice for filling out my survey.

The correct answer is carbohydrates.

Good nutritional understanding entails getting knowledge about what type of foods your body is expecting. From the beginning of time, there has been a tremendous amount of confusion about this. We have been told by society, advertising corporations, parents, and friends what our bodies should be consuming. And a great deal of the information that we have been given about this has been wrong.

In the predicament that human beings are in right now, with all of our health crises related to food, it's apparent that no one has been telling us the exact truth. If the exact truth was told and practiced, there would not be an epidemic of obesity, there would not be this much cancer, and there would not be as many people with dysfunctional digestive systems and other disorders. If humans were on the right path, these things would not be the case. But we are not on the right path.

65. Calories

In order for weight loss to occur, you must ultimately exert more energy than your caloric intake. This of course is one of the older paradigms of weight loss, and it works. However, most of what experts and laymen alike believe about calories is erroneous. In his book *The Calorie Myth*, Jonathan Bailor writes, "We regulate blood sugar with insulin injections. We track how many calories we eat and how many steps we take each day. We try to decipher food labels. We continue to get heavier and sicker while trying harder because the weight-loss prescription we've written is wrong."

If you can just restrict your calories, exercise a lot, never get cravings again, and never have any emotional setbacks, you'll be fine. You'll lose weight—it will just take time. Even if the food you eat is unhealthy, if your calories are low enough and your activity level is high enough then you've got to lose weight.

But this has nothing to do with total health. This has nothing to do with eating so that you have a low inflammatory diet to help reduce physical pain. This has nothing to do with eating so that you don't promote degenerative illnesses or cancer.

So calories are one factor. But they are one factor among many other important factors, such as eliminating processed food and reducing the amount of protein that you eat every day. You have to be cognizant of calories, but calories are not the most important thing regarding good overall health and a lasting lifestyle pattern in which weight control is a priority.

• •

The more you clean up your diet, the more biologically efficient your body becomes. The more efficient your body becomes, the more likely it is that you can consume a fair amount of calories and still drop some pounds.

• •

You could easily do an internet search and type in your height, your age, and your weight, plus a question about how many calories you need. Some diets have interactive apps that facilitate this. These programs are likely to put you into a calorie deficit of somewhere between 1500 and 1800 calories a day. On a standard Western diet, it's a fair assumption that a diet will be somewhere around 2000-2500 calories depending on the person's activity levels.

This doesn't take into account that a person doing a juice fast can be totally nourished and sustain a 1500 calorie per day diet for a very long period of time. And it doesn't take into account that if a person were to eat a 1500 calorie per day diet that consisted only of bacon, after about a month he or she would be on the brink of death.

A diet program that's teaching someone to understand their eating patterns won't just publish numbers to indicate how much a person may eat in a day. Some do practice diets based primarily on counting calories and they do very well. But most people fall short with such programs. And one reason that this is the case is that the problem is much more about what we eat than it is about how much we eat.

If we change our eating patterns, introduce wholesome foods, and allow our bodies to detox away from processed foods, our cravings will decrease and in turn we will eat less. If our diet consists of highly processed foods and junk foods, our cravings will soar. Subsequently we will eat more, our caloric intake will increase, we'll gain weight, and we'll feel terrible about it.

There are plenty of diets that you can go on that will crush your caloric intake as low as possible, enabling you to lose three pounds in a week. That's a struggle not worth the effort. You could lose two to three pounds in a week with the same caloric intake you had before just by doing the intermittent fasting program that I discuss later on in this book. Or you could lose two to three pounds in a week with the same caloric intake as in previous weeks by increasing your exercise activity dramatically. Or you could lose two to three pounds in a week with the same caloric intake by switching your diet to being 100% plant-based.

The second, third, and fourth weeks of a diet should be of great concern. What are you doing after the first week to make sure that you don't create a sluggish chemistry? Or if you're in a calorie deficit but are still eating processed food, you're likely to stumble into a chemically-based depression.

I have grave doubts about the long-term effects of diets focused on calorie counting and deficits. I've watched scores of people in my career start their diets carrying small scales with them and weighing their food. Sadly, many regained their weight after a time. Their ingrained unhealthy eating patterns didn't change over time.

The solution to weight control problems doesn't come in the form of an app or a pill. The solution comes in retraining your habits and dealing with your emotions. It comes in adapting a program that takes into account the way we think and feel about food and ourselves. It comes in dealing properly with our delicate and fragile emotional world. When we do that, we can withstand setbacks and not feel the need to self-destruct by using food to repress painful feelings.

The companies that are sending food to the house in portion meals are giving us a temporary solution, and this could be a good thing in the short run. If we can see the types of foods that we're supposed to be eating and then eat in a wholesome manner for a month or two, we might be able to interrupt our old unhealthy eating patterns. But remember, just getting a box of food sent to your door is not enough. You have to deal with emotional issues that are at the root of weight control problems, and you have to deal with those issues every day.

66. Protein

The adult body needs a small amount of protein, with extreme emphasis on the words "small amount." The amount is much less than what's been historically taught or recommended. And it's much, much less than the amount of protein we are accustomed to eating in the West.

People mistake the craving for protein as something healthy. But it isn't. The craving is similar to how we crave caffeine and feel relieved when we drink it. We become intoxicated by protein's effects; it provides us with a giant boost, and we don't feel right without it.

I am not surprised to be reminded that most people consider protein to be the most important nutrient. This is unfortunate for all of the creatures that have to donate their flesh.

We are not anatomically designed as carnivores. We do not have the eyesight, teeth, claws, speed, stealth, smell and digestive system to function optimally on a flesh-based diet.

• •

The idea that protein is a miracle nutrient is incorrect. And it's very important to realize that protein is not a weight loss solution that is either sustainable or healthy.

• •

The cells of your body make up the tissues of your body, which make up the organs of your body. Your body needs protein as a building block to form muscle, bone, and tissue. But once you are fully grown and living a normal active lifestyle, you don't need that much protein. Too much protein creates a problem in your chemistry—and it's not a solution to anything, especially weight loss.

My diet is low in protein compared to the diets of others. I do not crave protein any longer; I crave fruit and salads. It took me time and a better understanding of human chemistry to make the transition to where I am at now.

67. Carbohydrates

A statement made a few paragraphs ago bears repeating: The cells of your body make up the tissues of your body, which make up the organs of your body.

••

Humans need more protein during the growth years, when cells, tissues and organs are in their most formative stages. But humans need much less protein after they become fully grown adults. The nutrient (source of energy) that is then needed most is the carbohydrate—Prime Fuel #1.

••

We are primarily carbohydrate-burning machines. Any amateur nutritionist can validate this. Begging the question, what kind of carbohydrates? Answer: Vegetables and fruits.

All cells in your body move and carry out functions within your body using sugar molecules as fuel. That means everything you eat has to be converted, through chemical exchanges, into sugar.

••

All fruits are extraordinary fuel for humans. There are no bad fruits, and I have never met a single person in my life who struggles from fruit consumption. Fruit sugar is good sugar.

••

Any "expert" that steers you away from fruit has very limited experience and knowledge. Fruit should always be an integral part of a comprehensive health improvement program.

68. Fat

For some people, fat is an ugly word. We need dietary fats from the right foods, but certainly not from greasy food or processed sweets such as ice creams, cakes and candies. The healthiest source of dietary fat comes from plant sources. You do not need a single drop of fat (or protein for that matter) from an animal's body to subsist, and many forms of fat from animals bodies can be detrimental to our chemistry.

A ton of dietary misinformation and fad diets revolve around fat. These diets have temporary dramatic results but cause long-term detrimental results to your overall chemistry.

Following are some sources of good dietary fat:

Monounsaturated fat:

Olive, canola, rapeseed, peanut, and sesame oils	Avocados
Coconut meat	Olives
Unsalted nuts (almonds, peanuts, macadamia, hazelnuts, pecans, cashews)	Nut butters (almond or peanut butter)

Polyunsaturated fat:

Sunflower, sesame, and pumpkin seeds	Flaxseed
Walnuts	Fatty fish
Plant-based nut milks	Tofu, Tempeh, wheat gluten meat replacement products (I'm not a huge fan of these items; many of the commercial options are highly processed)

69. Vitamins and Minerals

We often put most of our concentration on the macronutrients: Carbohydrates, fats, and proteins. The reason is because they have calories and give us immediate energy.

The micronutrients come along with the macronutrients. To what degree depends on the type of food you are eating.

Foods like fruits and starchy vegetables (e.g., carrots) are where you'll find the greater density of vitamins. Vegetables (the leafy greens) are what have the greater density of minerals.

Fruits and vegetables—foods from the plant kingdom—are the purest source of food. When we eat the flesh of an animal or consume its eggs or animal secretions such as milk, we are getting the macronutrients and micronutrients but with the side effects of the impurities that live in the animal's body. When we take in those impurities, we need to get them out of our body.

The concerning impurities in the plant kingdom are the ones that humans pour into the environment. Be aware that all the flesh foods that we eat have these impurities as well. This is because all the animals we eat are made up of the substance that they acquired from their diet: Plants. According to scientificamerican.com, *a major problem in wild-caught fish are small particles of ingested plastic and the toxins they create. Farmed fish absorb toxins, as their environment contains land-based sources of pollution. Additionally, their primary feed source comes from conventionally grown terrestrial crops, which means that their diets can include trace amounts of pesticides and herbicides as well.*

Regarding micronutrients, we need far, far less of them than macronutrients to create the right interactions in the body. Everyone understands the basics about vitamins to some degree, as well as some basics about the immune system.

It's common knowledge that the immune system performs tasks that are separate from body functions performed by organs. And most people are aware that psychological events, stress, and other factors not associated with diet per se can have a negative effect on the immune system and subsequently on overall body health.

Much scientific evidence suggests that if people have emotional problems (even those caused by traumatic childhoods), those problems could be amplified by poor nutrition. The body and mind are linked in ways that science hasn't even begun to explain. So don't make light of the idea that if you're struggling with emotional problems that you should concentrate on the metaphorical lowest hanging piece of fruit (no pun intended). Specifically, that would be cleaning up your diet.

Having said that, diet cleanup is not a panacea. It will not fix all of your problems. But it is a very important part of a comprehensive program to achieve good health (including weight loss) and live life with more joy.

While you are on your journey of cleaning up your diet, you can benefit from taking high quality <u>supplements</u> that provide you with vital micronutrients.

The criteria for any supplement should be that the supplement manufacturer is comfortable with saying their product is 100% pure and unadulterated. If the claim is true, then you can be assured that the product isn't toxic in any way.

A good starting point for your supplement consumption would be a multivitamin (100% plant-based) and an effective plant-based probiotic. Everyone on earth can benefit from these two types of supplements.

After getting the basics, there's a plethora of supplements that may or may not be of help to you. But if the first criteria is met, you have nothing to lose but your money.

It can also be really valuable if you take a blood test and have it screened for vitamin deficiencies. But it would be a mistake to then run to the vitamin store and buy all those different vitamins and minerals. They would be less likely to work if your diet wasn't right.

Here is one example. Perhaps you are deficient in iron, and you run to purchase and then take a plant-based iron supplement. If you did so, you wouldn't have addressed the underlying problem. It could be that your thyroid improves when you use the supplement. However, the causation hasn't gone away—so another symptom will occur.

People tend to prefer buying things and taking them rather than working out whatever the problem is. The problem begins with the incorrect diet, exacerbated by stress and other deleterious lifestyle patterns such as lack of exercise and smoking tobacco.

70. Seasonal Foods

The issue of whether or not you should eat seasonal foods is an easy one. The answer is an emphatic yes. But if you live in places where the climate becomes freezing cold, you may be severely limited in your dietary choices. You will likely be forced to eat a lot of grains and flesh foods to maintain your body weight and to have energy to fulfill your activities.

It is a wonderful thing that in the modern world you can live in a place like Boston and still get delicious organic avocados in the winter. They're in season somewhere, even if it's winter in Boston. And it's fabulous that in the summertime you can drink coconut water in New York City, where coconuts don't grow. It's a blessing to consume açai berries and strawberries, almonds, grapes, peaches, nectarines, and so many other items even in the winter where you happen to be.

Most of us don't live off the land anymore—we rely on supermarkets. The supermarkets use distributors. The distributors use trucking, and the truckers are picking up things in Mexico to bring to New York City or Beverly Hills.

And we use boats to import seafood, coconuts, and so many other items. This giant economy and network of food circulation is a reality that we live in. In this book, it would be difficult to write about how to get off the grid, although I'd personally see that as an ideal way to live.

It would be a complex endeavor to have a farm that grew everything from olives to apples to avocados to red peppers to bell peppers to cucumbers to five or six different types of lettuces and to ginger.

But I'm not off the grid and I don't have farmland. And from the two or three experiences I had in growing things in my backyard, I understand it takes a lot of patience and effort to make sure that your produce survives to make it to your kitchen table.

71. You Are What You Eat—Eats

You are what you eat. And you are also what you eat—eats.

If you eat a cucumber, you are a cucumber. If you eat meat, you are the compounds that the meat consists of. But you are also what the animal eats, because that's what was in the animal's flesh at the time of its death. If your animal meal was fed byproducts and corn meal and antibiotics, then that's what you are.

....

If you desire to be a wholesome person, then eat wholesome foods, for God's sake.

....

It all makes perfect sense until you're out there in the world and your anxiety overwhelms you.

The reality that we live in pulls at our shirts. When our cravings kick in, we are not acting consciously anymore— we are just behaving in the way that is routine. Behaving routinely is comfortable, even if it is a path to destruction. It's how the human mind is set up; we are creatures of habit.

We are creatures of habit because we are not instinctual like other animals. We have to be taught how to live. Every detail. So when we find something that works and we make it into a pattern, that is what gives our conscious brain a sense of comfort.

Human beings are designed to eat the most nourishing foods that are energizing and stimulating early in the day, soon after or a little bit later than when we wake up. This sets us up for the most active time of the day.

(Unless you're doing intermittent fasting and your day starts at 12 noon, it's perfectly acceptable to live this way.) But the first foods that you eat will shape the rest of your day. At some point you're going to need calories from a clean source that has naturally occurring sugar in it.

This is so because that is the prime source of energy for human chemistry. If you eat things that are hard to digest or that are high protein, your body will feel sluggish by the middle of the day. Even if you've trained yourself to accept your being this way, you're sluggish compared to yourself (not compared to someone else). So, to reach your potential, the first meals of the day should be things that contain plenty of fresh fruit.

Frozen fresh fruit is a substitute for right off the vine fresh fruit, but it's still wonderful—especially in a smoothie, and of course if it's organic. And if you drink plenty of smoothies, it's best if you buy your produce fresh and freeze it yourself.

72. Consider Vegetarianism

I am a strong proponent of vegetarianism for quite a number of reasons. Complete vegetarianism may not be a realistic option for everyone. But at a minimum, all people—not just those concerned with weight loss—should focus their efforts on eating a great deal more fruits and vegetables and a great deal less animal protein.

To continue discussion of this particular topic, some historical, ideological, and sociological factors should be considered.

73. The Primary Food Sources: Humans Versus Other Animals

Any creature's features determine its likely primary food source. Human beings do not have claws, night vision, or a good sense of smell compared to other hunters. What we do have is adaptability and the capability to use tools, plus deep thinking that we can use to catch or grow our food.

Just because we can figure out how to catch a wild hog or salmon, this does not mean that the flesh material these creatures consist of is optimal for us. The mistake we make in our thinking is that just because we can eat these foods, we should. Just because we can eat a wide range of food groups does not mean that the particular foods are ideal.

Future historians will likely write the following regarding the previous 10,000 years to the present day: "Humans of that era were unconsciously eating because they did not know how to follow the instructions embedded in nature. They looked superficially at the objects they consumed with a lack of awareness as to the consequences their dietary mistakes had on their bodies and on their planet earth."

74. The Plant-Based Diet

The cleanest diet, the one that leaves the least amount of trash behind in the body chemistry, the one that is the most connected to the planet, is a plant-based diet. You are a carbohydrate-burning machine with a very long digestive system. Food that sits in your body for too long festers, and its festering causes all sorts of problems. To summarize—you were designed to eat plants, not flesh foods.

Flesh foods are secondary backup foods for different creatures such as humans and pigs when plant sources are scarce.

If there were no plant foods to be had, we could sustain life on flesh foods provided that we had 50% of our digestive system removed surgically. Sustaining life under such conditions would also require that you would have no stress in your life, that you would never breathe pollution, that you would always drink clean water, and that you would catch everything that you kill.

Animal protein is a cheat. It's a denser food because it's a concentration of material that is harder to digest. More calories are used to break down that fuel just to make it available for further energy. It is fuel that is squandered. Flesh foods have waste material in them that was present in the flesh of the animal, and your body has to remove it. On a molecular level, that flesh food contains compounds in excess that are toxifying and that make your body need to exert more energy to remove them.

• •

Plant-based foods such as vegetables, fruits, nuts, seeds, and sprouts are easily broken down by the human body. The nutrients that these plant-based foods contain subsequently become available for the body's use quickly. And there is very, very little waste material from plant foods, so the body doesn't have to expend much energy to remove what little waste those foods contain.

• •

The longer you eat a plant-based diet, the more you realize that fruit is necessary for energy. Without fruit, a person won't feel good, especially if they live an active lifestyle.

Fruit is extremely cleansing to a person's biological chemistry. Because fruit sugar is so easily absorbed and converted into fuel, it allows the body to focus on other tasks, including its own detoxification. Fruit sugar therefore fuels body detoxification.

Animal protein, on the other hand, is 50-75% waste material. Because this is so, your body must work harder to remove the generally nitrogenous byproducts of the meat that was eaten. This often includes the waste material that was in the animal, which must then be removed from your body as well.

Flesh foods may feel more filling and also may be more pleasurable to the senses. That is how you conditioned your senses. A meatball with tomato sauce may be more exciting to the tongue than an equal calorie amount of romaine lettuce. (That's not the case with me because for a long period of time I tuned out the meatball. But I do remember from many years ago how rich and heavy and luxurious it felt to eat that meatball.)

If I eat 300 calories of meatball versus 300 calories of salad, I become hungry about two times faster for more meatball and protein-rich foods than I do with the salad. That means to be comfortable I need to eat more calories if I eat flesh foods than if I eat plant foods. And that is why I gain weight; because I don't feel satisfied with an equal number of calories of flesh foods compared to plant foods.

The plant foods, calorie for calorie, simply have more compounds and nutrients that signal my chemistry as being full and happy in a way that flesh foods do not.

I took great pleasure in flesh-based foods for years and it took time to detox my senses for those foods. They may have indulged me but they did not fill me with the right substance for the life that I was then and am now trying to live: A diet with high integrity and great consciousness, one that promotes my maximum health and does not run me out of vitality, a diet that is also sensitive to the suffering and murdering of countless animals.

I want to be clear—I'm not trying to convince you to be a vegan. That lifestyle is not for everyone—but I won't back down from the stance that universally, regardless of what we may be told, it is the best diet for humans. And I recommend that everyone consider it.

You may be aware of all the difficulties that some vegans who go back to eating meat have encountered. I've experienced them myself. I had times during my own journey when I felt hungry. I had emotional things going on in my life, I was very active, and I wasn't eating the right diet. I didn't have the proper balance of nutrients, so I had cravings for heavy foods. At times those cravings were overwhelming.

There were times in my diet when I would see a piece of fish with a salad and I wanted to tackle the bowl of salad and eat the hand of the person eating it. I was so hungry. But I had made a commitment to a certain diet because I understood it was the right thing for me to do, and so I had to go through those difficult stages.

But once you clearly understand that detoxifying yourself from a certain lifestyle and pattern is a process, and that you are on the right mission, it's not as frightening or depressing to go through the rough times.

Again, I am not attempting to convert all my readers into vegetarians. I'm just trying to tell the truth about serious dietary mistakes, most or all of which I've made myself. And I'm even going to help readers continue to eat flesh-based foods if that is what they deeply desire to do. But my hope is that over time readers will become willing to let go of all their dietary errors.

Being vegan and eating clean is not a panacea for all that ails you. You can eat a great diet yet still become ill because there are so many components to your chemistry. But this is no excuse to say, "What the f**k, I've got to live my life, so I'm going out for pasta and meatballs at 11:30, and then I might as well polish off that bottle of wine."

Rather than that, putting yourself on a path toward good dietary health and sticking to it, despite temptations and difficulties, is what you need to do.

75. Good Plant Foods and Where to Find Them

It is true that supermarkets and other retail stores aggressively market unhealthy foods. But although that's the case, you're not deprived of good food choices at this time in the West. You have hundreds of plant-based, all natural, unprocessed choices available. It may be necessary to go to reputable health food and similar stores for some items, but if you're careful and selective you can find good options even at your local supermarket or wholesale club.

These vegetables and others should be available in the produce section: romaine lettuce, parsley, red leaf lettuce, boston lettuce, green leaf lettuce, radishes, carrots, scallions, celery, parsnip, beets, cilantro, kale, collard greens, bok choy, broccoli, cauliflower, cabbage, chives, plantains, asparagus, zucchini, eggplant, red peppers, green peppers, and corn.

These fruits and nuts and many others should be available in the produce section: lemons, oranges, honeydew melon, kiwi, bananas, tangerines, watermelon, avocado, coconut, cashews, and almonds.

76. I Am Obsessed With Fruits, Vegetables, Nuts, Sprouts, and Seeds

My diet is 100% plant-based. I love fruits, vegetables, nuts, and produce. I drink a very small amount of espresso coffee in the morning.

I love every single vegetable on planet earth that is edible to humans. I like to eat them raw, and I like to eat them cooked. I highly recommend a plant-based diet.

Should you decide to adapt a largely or wholly plant-based diet, think of your vegetable and fruit diet as if you were a child and you had a playroom. The more variety of toys you have, the more interesting the room is to you. Ask yourself this question: "When was the last time I ate a carrot, some celery, a cucumber or two, radishes, olives, walnuts, cherries, peaches, apples, pineapple, avocado, red peppers, green peppers, or beets?"

The more extensive that your dietary bouquet of colors and textures from the plant kingdom is, the more complete and the more precise your diet will be. You will be incorporating into your diet a variety of compounds that will restore and protect the body's systems.

If you're starting a plant-based diet, I recommend that you commit yourself to 30 days of 100% uncooked vegetables and fruits. Go through the experience. It may make you gaseous or tired at first, but I advise gutting it out just to prove to yourself that you can subsist on nothing more than fruit and vegetables. They don't have to be fried, baked, sautéed, or microwaved; they can just be eaten raw.

Some people might ask, "What about my thyroid problem or my diabetes?" By all means seek competent medical advice under such circumstances. I can't give you any advice because that would create liability for me, but I will say that you should not be fearful of uncooked fruits and vegetables.

Do not drink alcohol during the 30-day period, and eat 100% raw food from plants only.

••

You must rid yourself of the faulty thinking that you will die without processed food and/or animals and animal products.

••

After your 30 days, you can begin to add things back into your diet and see how you feel. Of course if you were addicted to Hostess Twinkies before, and after 30 days you had a Hostess Twinkie, I'd guess that you'd feel a lot better for pandering to the sugar craving. But that feeling of goodness would be deceptive. Don't eat the Twinkie.

This would be similar to the situation of people who inject heroin into their arms. They feel psychologically better but don't care about the harmful effects of the drug. Although most of us are not drug addicts, it takes us a long time to detox from heavily processed foods, refined sugar, and other products that made us feel safe even though they were unhealthy.

The human body can heal itself miraculously. If you have a good diet, you will experience changes in your body chemistry. Given time, your chemistry will change to cause you to be at the exact weight that you should be. Your chemistry will be different from the body chemistry of an overweight person. The chemistry will affect your mood and your thinking, changing it for the better.

77. Water and Hydration

No book on diet would be complete if it didn't cover the subject of water and hydration to some degree. In order for your system to function correctly, you have to be well hydrated. You have latitude and a tolerance for plus or minus, too much or too little water in your system at any given time. But when you live outside of this tolerance you will be out of balance. That includes everything—your metabolic functions, your sense of well being, your immune system, recovery, energy levels, and so much more.

There are a number of aspects of water that are critical to the weight loss process. One aspect is how important it is to your chemistry to have a proper balance of $H2O$ in your system. It's necessary so that your chemistry will be able to process the foods that you eat and maintain homeostasis and balance.

Hunger elicits a sensation of physical pain. And for most of us, when we feel that type of pain we feel an accompanying sense of anxiety. This anxiety is a trigger for acting out negatively (including overeating or eating junk food). The part of your brain that controls hunger is called the hypothalamus.

Your blood sugar levels also tell your brain that you are running low on food. Oftentimes our consciousness relates some of the pains that we feel in our stomach with hunger pangs. But at times these may actually be gas pains. When you are cleaning up your diet, it's very common for gases to release various pressures from your overall system. In a sense, you are deflating.

Your stomach tells your brain that you are full. That's why it's important that your first reaction to hunger should be to drink water. It signals your brain that you are not in danger. It should also help you determine the time you need to plan your meal.

Like food, your drinking water should be pure. It's a crying shame that we have to drink bottled water coming from other regions. But we won't spend time right now complaining about this environmental condition.

In the context of this book, water is considered an essential nutrient because it is required in amounts in excess of what we can produce on our own. So in essence water and air are two completely overlooked critical nutrients. This is the case because when people think of nutrients they think soley of food.

Our chemistry will certainly be out of whack if we aren't breathing consciously throughout the day, or if we restrict breathing because of tension and stress. It will also be out of whack if we deprive ourselves of water for any reason.

Reaching out for clean water is one of the first and most vital self-healing activities. We have been rightfully taught that from early childhood. We are taught very young to reach for a water bottle and explore the texture. We love to play in water as children, both because it is a powerful metaphor of the emotions and because playing in water is fun.

Make sure that you drink plenty of water every day as part of your weight loss regimen. The amount of water that we need varies in different stages of our lives and also based on which sex we are. It's easy to research exactly how much water you need to consume based on your age, your weight, and your activity level. In general, women need about 11 1/2 cups per day and men need about 15 1/2 cups per day.

Remember that you also get a significant amount of water from the food you eat. Eating plump fruits is incredibly beneficial, not only for the nutrients that they provide but also for the water that they contain.

A little-known secret about the body is that if the back of the throat is dry, it will signal your brain that you're hungry when in fact you're only thirsty. So make sure you keep your mouth wet with water throughout the day. This is a valuable tip for both weight loss and overall body health.

You already know that it's essential to drink water in order to not die, but what you might not know is that water helps your chemistry achieve the dropping of unnecessary weight. Lowering your caloric intake and increasing your physical activity is not enough. There are other chemical and biological processes that are completely dependent on the right amount of water being present in order to facilitate weight loss.

But that's not all. Water is the ultimate medium for the transmission of invisible data. Our knowledge and our emotions are carried through this conductive material. So it is important that you realize that there's such a thing as junk food water that's low in energy, low in frequency, and low in vibration. It leaves us thirsty and dehydrated. So it goes without saying that the quality of the water we drink will determine the quality of our overall bodily composition (which of course includes our emotional composition).

In this book I'm not going to embark on any hippie dippy stuff and tell you how to charge water with crystals. But I'm going to say that you have to make time in your day to provide yourself with water. It should be the case that the first sensation of abundance and prosperity that you will feel each day is that of being properly hydrated.

When you're dehydrated, the body signals the consciousness that there is danger or trouble. We can be so accustomed to the feeling that we don't even know what the source of it is. So please drink a boatload of water. Seriously: Drink the appropriate amount for your activity level and your body size.

Make sure that your water is very pure. Do not compromise on the purity of your water. Municipal tap water is sh*t. It's filled with compounds that even the best filter systems cannot get rid of. When people put reverse osmosis water filters in their home, those systems have to be accompanied with remineralization agents. It's a giant mess.

The politics of water are beyond the scope of this book. But give it some thought. Your happiness and your health are inextricably linked to the substance of water. What do you actually know about it? What do you truly know about the bottled water you're drinking? What are the processes and practices of the facilities that are bottling the water that you put into your body?

Please pay close attention: I recommend that the first thing that you do after you wake up and perhaps say a few words of gratitude is to reach for clean drinking water and fill up. In order for me to remember to drink water I have two key times of the day that I load up. When I wake up, before I do anything, I drink water until I feel like I'm drowning. I do so again in the middle of the day.

Those are my two big pit stops. I personally do not like to hydrate too much an hour or so before bedtime, because it'll wake me up. But I do sip water throughout the night before bedtime, because a dry throat is a distraction. And any thirst might deceive my mind into thinking that I'm hungry.

Here's a little tidbit that makes this discussion of water totally worthwhile: Your brain likely doesn't really know the difference between hunger and thirst. Sometimes when the body is signaling hunger, the body might actually just be thirsty. So it's good if you're at a calorie deficit and you feel hungry to just drink some water.

Also, thirst and hunger begin in the back of the throat. If the throat is poorly hydrated and becomes dry, the brain is signaled that something is going on that needs our attention. We can easily misinterpret the dry throat communication because we've lost our primordial connection to all such communications.

So we might eat or feel the anxiety of hunger when we may have just been thirsty. We can mistake a parched dry throat as our body saying, "Oh my God, I'm starving!" Just moisten the back of the throat with a good chug of clean water. This will give you some time to figure out whether or not you're hungry and respond without panic.

Invest some time in learning about issues pertaining to water purity. Water now is one of our very highly processed "foods." I believe that even the healthiest people don't do enough to avoid municipal water that has synthetically-made fluoride added to it. Your amazing home filter, unless it is distilling or doing reverse osmosis, doesn't get rid of fluoride. Municipal water also contains chlorine, pharmaceutical waste, a host of bacteria, and other toxic materials.

Don't get nervous: Really amazing clean spring water is available to you in the bottle. I am concerned about the 5 gallon bottles that are used and reused, though. I'm concerned about what they clean those reusable containers with. I am not hypervigilant, but I do think about these things.

Drinking bottled water is a tiresome and expensive habit. Not everyone can afford the luxury of building out a multi-stage, comprehensive household water filter system. In the large kitchen that I built for Juice Press, I had the pleasure of participating in the engineering of incredible water filtration systems.

If you are going to filter your home, I would just filter the drinking water system. But I don't like the reverse osmosis system. It is extremely wasteful and it demineralizes the water, which becomes a problem over the long run.

The filtration systems that can remove fluoride and some other really nasty microbes rely on charred animal bone as the medium to capture those chemical compounds. If you have the time and the patience to do extensive research, you can get yourself set up with an incredible filter system that takes out a lot of the things you don't want in your body. I assure you that in a short period of time you will feel better from just this one thing—clean drinking water.

In the future I believe that we will have good leadership in all levels of government, and repair of our vital water supplies will become a priority. Let this be the beginning of that discussion for you. Right now, though, be self-centered and only care about the quality of the water that you're putting in your body. Try not to be lured in by whoever has the best packaging. You will need to exercise discernment and involve yourself in the study of this somewhat complex subject—it is of paramount importance to you and your loved ones.

78. Fall in Love With Salad

When in doubt, eat a green salad. And throw some other vegetables and fruits in there, like tomatoes and red peppers. Teach yourself how to make a good salad dressing. Or if you're lazy, there are salad dressings out there that are USDA Organic with clean ingredients. My favorite company is Bragg. Their products taste good and are very wholesome. But nothing beats the salad dressing made by you at home.

You don't just pour salad dressing on the salad and then shove it down your throat. If you make a good salad dressing, it's really a marinade designed to pre-digest your leaves. So you should rub the salad dressing into the leaves and let it sit for 15 minutes before you eat it.

The middle of the day is a great time for a salad. I recommend eating your largest, most filling meal in the middle of the day. This is because your body is still awake and you still have time to utilize extra energy.

Humans can actually live on salad alone, as long as there is enough diversity of produce from day to day and as long as the salads have enough calories. If grains and animal protein are added, they should be eaten with large leafy green salads.

Some people hate vegetables. Perhaps you hate vegetables more than anything else in this world. I really feel for you if your appetite is set up that way—I'm terribly sorry that that's the case. But I have a hard time imagining any other creature that wouldn't be disgusted by what the ordinary human diet is.

I make that statement just as a bit of fun. And perhaps I'm being judgmental by making it. I'm very aware that I'm not the perfect person to describe how to fix that aspect of your diet.

You probably know that science is in my favor regarding dangers of flesh-based foods. Medical people tell those with digestive illnesses to reduce fat intake, processed food, and cow's milk, and they also tell them to eat more fruits and vegetables, including leafy greens.

Doctors have been giving advice along these lines since the 1970s. Before that, it was likely that the doctor told such people to eat more chicken versus red meat and to switch from eating white bread to eating whole wheat bread. That was pretty much the extent of the good dietary advice that the medical community gave to the people at the time.

Over the last 50 years, the world has been getting more overweight than ever before, and I don't profit from this. The last thing I want to see is other people suffering. I'm also trying to help you to make the connection between bad dietary choices and people suffering.

But I remember a lot of years of just simply being in denial. There was nothing that anyone could tell me to make me hear something that I didn't want to hear. It was likely because I wasn't ready to change, or because I disagreed, or both. I didn't disagree because I had a deep level of knowledge. I just knew what my cravings were but I didn't want the discomfort of not listening to all of my impulses and urges.

It's uncomfortable for a person, especially a person with lots of anxiety, to have urges that they can't fulfill and cravings that they can't satiate. But I have to tell you the truth about these matters, and I also hope to share my experience, strength, and hope with you.

When I was involved with my company (Juice Press) for approximately 10 years, I taught hundreds of thousands of people throughout New York City and other major cities to enjoy the delicious taste of fresh, cold-pressed organic juice. When you drink juice you get a lot of produce without having to gag on it, and it tastes great, but only if it's very cold. (If you drank juice from really dark, leafy green vegetables at room temperature you probably wouldn't like it.) That's the beauty of cold-pressed juice—the cold temperature makes it taste great, like a smoothie. Certain foods taste better at different temperatures; I think pasta only tastes good when it's warm.

So, if you're thinking that it's really important for you to get more dark, hard-to-eat leafy greens into your system, think about blending them into smoothies and mixing them up with something sweet. For example, you could have a berry smoothie with bananas and put tons of fresh spinach in it. Add some ice cubes and some dates or other fruits. Whole fruits that are not processed are best.

You will get sugar from the fruit. Because the sugar isn't refined, it isn't going to wreak havoc on your chemistry the way that processed, refined sugar does. In some of my other articles, I give details regarding how refined sugar affects your chemistry; the chemistry behind it is actually very simple.

In conclusion, if you're having a hard time getting used to leafy greens and even cruciferous vegetables like broccoli, please get yourself a blender and a juice machine. It's so easy to create the lifestyle pattern of getting good nutrition from vegetable juices. For the first couple of months you may kick and scream. You will have to do cleanup and you'll have to buy things. But the tremendous payoff will be that you'll feel fantastic and you'll get healthier.

Having the ability to make juices and smoothies at home will definitely mean that you'll make better choices more than half the time. They'll be an immediate improvement in your chemistry every time you do so. Metaphorically speaking, your body will forgive you right away for every sin that you might have committed. This will happen because you repented of your dietary error, did something healthy, and engaged in positive thinking while you were in the process.

79. Fall in Love With Juices and Smoothies

I am the world's most excited proponent of all fresh, raw juices. I owned more than 85 juice bars at one time!

Your body is expecting lots of leafy greens of varied kinds. For that reason and others, I rely heavily on greens and green juices.

I drink at least 16 ounces per day of fresh raw green juice. If such juice is not available, I have a very pure USDA organic superfood powder that I mix into water. I like how it makes me feel—very strong and healthy.

•••

A chemical fact that many laymen and even professionals do not quite understand is as follows: Because of the extremely high mineral content in the detoxification process, it is apparent that the minerals in the greens are pulling carbonic acid and other toxic compounds from the cells. Simply put, ingesting greens helps us release toxins.

•••

Eating a mostly raw diet is not an easy feat to accomplish. It is the ultimate diet, and the most controversial. There are many aspects of it that are difficult to explain or understand if you haven't experienced them personally.

The time a detoxification process takes depends on the individual's body chemistry and a number of other circumstances. When beginning a raw food diet, a person will often feel worse before they feel better.

They may feel as if they are making mistakes, but actually they are cleansing their bodies. If they eat some cooked foods, instead of being completely raw, they create a margin of error. If you are 80% raw, but drink plenty of fresh juice and have a positive attitude, you can be unbelievably healthy and live a supreme life.

People must understand that there is more to healthy eating than simply counting calories. Although the body is a powerhouse when it comes to healing and detoxification, it is each person's responsibility to ensure that what they eat aids the body in those cleansing, healing, and detoxification processes.

It is best to consume greens early in the day, but fruit can be consumed at any time. Fruit and food combinations are extremely important, and become much more critical when more food is being consumed at once. These combinations are less critical when people eat smaller meals, but proper food combinations should still be followed in order to avoid fermentation, which can lead to inflammation.

Getting your vegetables from fresh, raw juices is totally 1000% acceptable and amazing in every way. Especially with a plant-based diet, because you need far less fiber than you do when you consume a fair amount of meat, fish, chicken, or other animal proteins.

Juices are healthy in every way; do not be afraid of them. Make juice at home or find a place that makes cold-pressed juices fresh every day. All produce should be USDA certified organic. Pay attention to expiration dates. Juice that has not been pasteurized in any way should have a shelf life of 2-3 days.

Juices that are pasteurized last far longer than juices that have not been treated. But I am strongly against the HPP process of preserving juices. First and foremost, they taste absolutely nasty. Additionally, they are not cheaper than fresh juices and they have diminished nutrient and enzyme values. The bad taste alone should be reason enough to opt for fresh juices instead.

I am also a massive fan of hand-crafted organic smoothies, with emphasis on freshly made and zero bad ingredients. Where can you get those? There are not too many places that have high quality ingredients and that do not cut corners. Most smoothie places do not have a real health program.

The base of a smoothie is the liquid. It (as well as the other ingredients) should be made daily and with no sweeteners added. And no emulsifiers or thickening agents should be used. The commercial liquids used at smoothie places are industrially made and pasteurized.

You want the best organic superfood and protein powders made from plants for purity and zero inflammation response. Avoid the heck out of whey protein. Frozen fruits must all be frozen when ripe. Use organic ingredients or only shop at organic smoothie bars. It's an integral part of a true health paradigm. No pesticides and USDA Organic labeling will indicate better handling practices in general.

Make smoothies at home for the best results. Cleaning up is far easier than juicing. Frozen fruit is easier to deal with. Smoothies are meal replacements and I think they are optimal for breakfast or lunch. Be courageous with plant-based ingredients.

Avoid filling your smoothie with caffeinated products, unless you really need to. But even then, please don't. Stimulation accelerates the aging process. Always. I love adding fresh ginger to a smoothie, as well as cinnamon, cardamon, almond butter, blue-green algae, probiotics, and anything else that's plant-based and yummy.

80. Development in Human Diet Patterns

Eating plants for ancient humans was experimental. They learned from their mistakes. The knowledge about successful and unsuccessful plant-eating practices was passed on from one generation to another.

Relying on other beasts for our fuel has always been a safe gamble. It was easy to structure a society as being flesh food based. When we are all hungry and we cook up some beef, we will all go to bed satiated (at least in the short run).

Culturally, flesh foods (e.g., red meat, poultry, fish, dairy, eggs, and insects) were an easy choice. They seemed to pose a lower immediate risk of danger of sickening the body. As an example, people realized that eating poison berries could kill you. It took time to figure out what was and what wasn't poison in the plant kingdom. With flesh foods, things were generally less complicated—kill a creature, cook it and eat it, and it's not likely to be poisonous if it's stored and cooked properly.

Plant foods initially would require greater skill to find, plant, grow, harvest and prepare. With plant foods, a wider range of material (variety of produce and plant food groups) was required to give clan members a sense of being full. More plant material was required for the comparable amount of calories in flesh foods.

The flesh diet mentality must be derived from a society that has as one of its core beliefs that one beast is meant to be a slave to another. Many members of our society do not think this deeply about food. They follow the herd, and in whatever direction the herd moves, they follow without question.

A society seeking peace can't be built upon the blood and suffering of any other type of creature. This has nothing to do with heaven and hell—there should be no fire and brimstone preaching in connection with this issue. Creatures who live desire life more than anything else.

This is why the flesh-based diet is not ideal for humans. We are the highest order of creatures in this realm. For our development, we are required to master compassion; this is what opens our consciousness to deeper levels of understanding about creation and everything else.

Eating is linked to your deepest origins, including your society and your ideas regarding God. For you to have proper ideas about weight loss, you need to have an understanding of these particular concepts.

81. Cow's Milk and Chicken Eggs

You have noted that throughout this book I speak quite negatively and in no uncertain terms about dietary mistakes such as eating processed foods.

I'm certain that I would sell a lot more copies of this book if the program said that you could eat lots of Oreo cookies and not exercise. Or that if you took a certain pill and refrain from eating kumquats anymore that you'd shed pounds in record time.

I clearly understand the science behind matters of diet and lifestyle. And I understand that certain things have to be eliminated completely from your diet in order for you to achieve overall success.

In light of that, I must stress the importance of eliminating dairy products, especially dairy products from cows. This is very difficult for those vegetarians who really enjoy milk products. But there are problems associated with milk, which I will explain.

Milk is unquestionably a miraculous substance. It contains the critical nutrients to nurture newborns and help them continue to grow in all vital ways outside of the womb of the mother. Brain development, organ development, bone growth, muscle growth, and the central nervous system all have to grow rapidly in the first couple of years of life.

Human mother's milk is designed to take a 6-8 pound infant at birth to approximately 30 pounds by age three. There are compounds in all animals' mother's milk that induce growth. A cow weighs an average of 86 pounds at birth. By the time the calf is weaning, that calf's weight is approximately 600 pounds.

The raw compounds in cow's milk are too growth-inducing for human chemistry. The elements are much too overstimulating for the human body, and such overstimulation causes irritation in a child's body.

The body's response mechanism to such irritation is to create an inflammatory immune response. Under that level of irritation, the body will also secrete mucus in a variety of places. It will do so as a protective response to the inflammation caused by the compounds in the milk—specifically, the naturally occurring growth hormones such as casein.

Milk from a cow is not bioidentical to the milk from a human being. And it's also an issue that a grownup usually isn't trying to grow larger. By drinking milk, adults are just drinking a substance that will make them feel full but with the side effect of creating mucus and inflammation.

To make matters worse, cows are no longer natural organic creatures. Female cows are injected with hormones to keep them producing milk far longer than they would be doing otherwise. The chemistry of cows bred for producing dairy products is completely out of whack. They are loaded with growth-inducing hormones and other chemicals. Those chemicals are passed along to anyone who drinks the milk from those cows.

To make matters worse, the cows we are drinking milk from are miserable. They are stationary, and in order to keep them from getting sick from the horrendous conditions they live in, they are given large doses of antibiotics. Antibiotics are compounds that kill bacteria—both good and bad. So those who drink milk are also getting an antibiotic treatment, even if it's diluted and muted to some degree.

There is a cheat to cow's milk, and I'm hesitant to offer it. I don't do it myself, but I'll offer it anyway, in the hope that I will sell more books. If you have to eat a dairy product to keep from losing your mind, consume the milk from much smaller animals that are nearly identical to the size and the weight of a human, such as sheep and goats.

Also, only use cheese that is rennet-free. I will explain that substance in another book. If you eat aged cheese made of sheep or goat's milk, then the naturally occurring hormones will be less potent due to the aging process of the cheese. Again, these tips are cheats of sorts. You can do fine without dairy products altogether if you choose to.

I know that what stays on the minds of many people is the image of the beautiful blonde running up a hill with two pails of milk, and she looks like a goddess. And we sometimes reflect on all the people around the world who've done quite well with dairy as part of their diets, and that confuses us.

But we're not looking at the whole picture. She may have looked spectacular at 18 but far less so at 39. Diet plays a huge part in how quickly we accelerate our aging.

We also have to take into consideration what her overall diet and lifestyle might have been. It's likely that the young maiden living on the hill in the 19th century was breathing clean air. It's likely that she was also drinking uncontaminated water. And she would not have had access to the abominable concoctions that are today's processed foods. Since she would not have had those things working against her, her margin for dietary error would have been huge.

If you contrast that idyllic scenario to that of the modern-day individual who lives in a big city and shops at giant supermarkets, the outcome isn't pretty. Our modern-day diet and lifestyle is filled with pollution, too much stress, questionable water sources, heavily processed food products, heavy reliance on protein, and many little chemistry mistakes floating around in the background. With so little margin for error, the dietary mistake of consuming dairy products is too overwhelming for the body.

Over a span of 10 years, I talked to a huge number of people when I was immersed in customer relations at Juice Press. I told many of them to simply eliminate dairy from their diet. Many of them did nothing else but eliminate dairy and lost 15 to 20 pounds in two or three months. And some others experienced far less or no arthritis pain just by eliminating dairy.

At this point, I want to make it clear that I am addressing adult dietary needs in this book. A child's needs are considerably different from those of an adult. So I'm not giving recommendations about what children should subsist on. Although I fully believe in the vegan diet for children, it's a much harder diet for children to adhere to for social and other reasons that I won't go into in this book. So, again, the diet that I espouse pertains to adults.

How about eggs? Egg whites were extremely popular when I was a teenager. I'd eat about 15 of them a day to get protein for stronger muscles. I had no idea what I was doing to the rest of my chemistry, particularly regarding the burden I was placing on my liver.

I did consult with my food mentor and some friends with PhDs about this matter. For the most part, they collectively agreed that two or three eggs per week from clean free range animals not pumped up with antibiotics wouldn't be harmful to those observing the various dietary improvements detailed in this book.

The best way to cook an egg is to not fry it in oil. Poached eggs and hard-boiled eggs are best. If you are transitioning away from an animal-based diet, then eggs might help make the transition easier. You don't need to eat them every day, though: Doing so is not recommended.

One other thing: As I've stated before, any time you consume animal protein it's best not to eat it alone. It's better to eat it with a large leafy green salad.

82. Don't Let Pious Vegans Judge You

Throughout this book I make statements about animal proteins that are based on science. Specifically, on the science of anatomy and the science of chemistry. I'm not preaching a vegan diet to the world at this time. It so happens that I am 100% plant-based. But it took me many years to get to this point, and two things in particular helped me make the transition.

The first thing was that I needed to lose weight and keep it off. I discovered through my trainers that a plant-based diet would be the very best way for me to maintain an extremely low body weight during my fighting years. The motivation to succeed in that realm gave me a tremendous boost.

The second impetus came later. At that point in time I had started a chain of plant-based restaurants. Many customers and other people were scrutinizing me and my diet. I became very self-conscious, and this motivated me to get as close to dietary perfection as possible.

Also, because I owned those restaurants, I was able to just walk down the block from my apartment to one of them. I could grab a smoothie, a juice, a salad, or one or more of many kinds of vegan snacks and treats. This made it very easy for me to eat well all the time. I didn't have to shop, wash produce, prepare anything, or clean up the kitchen. The plant-based lifestyle was effortless for me.

I realize now that entering into a vegan lifestyle has its hurdles. One of the hurdles entails juggling our emotions. We must juggle feelings of hunger and fears that we are not getting enough protein, vitamins, and minerals, with the moral dilemma of slaughtering animals for food. It's a lot to deal with all at once.

But I want the program that I'm writing about to be accessible to as many people as possible. I don't want people to say that there's good stuff in this book but that the overall program is too hard.

So please don't feel judged by anyone if you choose to eat animal protein. I know that you can be extremely healthy consuming flesh foods as long as you do it in a way that your body can deal with. You don't have to be a vegan to be extremely healthy—that's a fact. You just have to consume flesh foods mindfully and skillfully.

First and foremost, do not eat more than three servings of animal protein in a 7-day period of time. Flesh foods are defined as red meat, white meat, fowl, fish, aquatic mammals, turtles, snails, squirrels, snakes, and other animals. This also includes the eggs of these animals. And please note that honey is not a flesh food.

If you do consume animal protein, do so a maximum three times a week, every other day at most. **Always eat flesh foods with a large leafy green salad.** The salad is the correction and the fiber needed to push hard to digest substances like flesh through the digestive system. In theory, the salad is a true digestive aid.

True carnivores eat the entire body of their prey. The lucky ones get to the entrails of the animal that they are eating. The entrails contain lots of undigested plants. The carnivore is eating the flesh of the animal with a delicious salad. I have a theory, unproven as of yet, that carnivores would probably live longer if humans fed them blended salad smoothies every day.

My mentor taught me that with a large leafy green salad you can cover up most dietary mistakes, within reason. Here's the recap: (1) always eat animal protein with a large leafy green salad; (2) don't gluttonize and eat 16-ounce steaks; (3) don't combine flesh foods with starchy carbohydrates such as potatoes, rice or bread (in other words, the sandwich itself is a huge dietary mistake); and (4) don't eat fruit either one hour before or one hour after eating flesh foods.

With the above things taken into consideration, it may sound as if you have just gotten a pass to eat flesh foods for the rest of your life. But under some circumstances, a person should consider not having flesh foods at all. This is the case with people who have certain illnesses or diseases that they are trying to heal from. Those with cancer and inflammatory diseases, especially inflammatory diseases of the digestive system, will do 1000% better immediately if they adopt a plant-based diet.

The next consideration for being able to consume flesh foods safely is to really understand the sources of those foods. Livestock that is raised indoors—animals that barely see sunlight, do not have an opportunity to move freely, are kept in stalls, fed corn and animal byproducts, and are pumped with hormones to accelerate their growth processes—is an abomination of our food supply.

Raising animals in this way should not be legal. It is absolute horrible torture to these thinking and feeling creatures, and that should be the primary consideration for choosing not to consume these animals. But in addition to that, the processes of raising these animals are extremely corrupting and destructive to the substances that these flesh foods consist of.

It is imperative that we go after ethically sourced, sustainably raised, clean animal-based food. It may be more expensive, but objection to the price is the wrong way of looking at this. It's not that it's more expensive—it's that these types of animal-based foods are praiseworthy. Foods should be praised in this day and age. The things that are cheaper are produced using despicable cheats. The cheats are not only terrible for the animals, they're awful for the planet and they're destructive to your body chemistry.

To summarize, the major considerations of your diet should be to not eat too much animal protein and to eliminate processed food and other dietary mistakes (which are discussed throughout this book). The most difficult thing may be just the idea of separating from flesh foods, because such foods stimulate us and make us feel full.

I don't want the thought of complete abstinence from flesh foods to be an obstacle in your path at this point in your recovery. Later on, as you stabilize from addictive eating patterns, you can consider going on to the more advanced things that are suggested. It also might be helpful for you to start competitively fighting and opening up your own chain of juice bars. (LOL)

83. Ethical Considerations

Unfortunately, all the processes that can make a compound can also have bad side effects. Food and medicines in their natural forms communicate with the body chemistry in a positive way; that's what we're looking for in a diet. We're looking for food sources that have not been perverted and corrupted. We're looking to eat things that are truly compassionate to the world outside of us and the chemistry inside of us. I consider this concept to be scientific rather than spiritual.

If I eat foods that require brutality, how could that brutality not energize, materialize, and be transfered into my body and my very being? Even if it's subtle and unconscious to me, if I consume animals, I have to be eating all the terror, fear, sorrow and anger that was experienced by that animal.

I have been a plant-only eater for quite some time, but I realize that that's a difficult menu to follow for most people. But I highly recommend it, not only for your body chemistry but for your spiritual and emotional growth as well. Many meat eaters may be spiritually, emotionally, and ethically way ahead of me, but I cannot recommend eating the flesh of an animal because it doesn't suit me. I also think it's a benefit to the creatures on the planet that if you find it necessary to continue to eat flesh-based foods, you do so conscientiously.

For example, you can make a choice to eat free range chickens. If that's the case, you should be able to verify a number of things. Do the chickens live on a farm running free? Do they know there's a building structure over there to the far right with machines that dismember them and prepare them for their journey to the consumers' mouths?

Cows that live in the open pasture, grazing all day, farting and talking to their cousins and uncles, will definitely give out a few angry moos when they're prodded onto a truck to go to the slaughterhouse. But the main thing is if they lived a somewhat natural life in a field and were cared for, that energy will be in their bloodstream.

Some will argue that wild-caught fish live free until they're pulled up on a boat. But there's something slightly backwards in the logic of "fishing for pleasure." There's no fish that enjoys having a hook put in its mouth, and then sitting in a storage bin on ice for a couple of days with hundreds of other fish crashing down on it while it suffocates to death.

Just be aware of this. Put it into your consciousness in the event that there may be a time you get tired of being a part of that unconscious feeding loop. I cannot judge you, because at one point in my life I ate meat as well. But there should not be any confusion about the fact that we do not need meat to survive.

It doesn't matter what you're told on wrappers of food products, on the Oprah Winfrey show, or in 3-inch-thick books on nutrition. Probably more than 95% of those with PhDs or medical licenses don't understand the chemistry of nutrition any better than you will by the time you finish this book.

There's clear evidence regarding nutrition all around us. And we can't rely on the government to safely guide us, despite their good intentions, because of the enormous bureaucracy within the Food and Drug Administration.

But I would be extremely impressed if the FDA published information on how to successfully be a vegan. The science on veganism is clear and shows that vegans have far less degenerative illness than others. Yet vegans can be unhealthy people if they eat junk foods and such; guidance is necessary.

Although the purpose of this book is not to "preach veganism," I hope that the content does cause you to consider it as an option. One should think deeply about the situation that creatures capable of feeling pain must die in order that we may be fed.

84. Alcohol, Tobacco, Inhaling Smoke From Cannabis, and Other Drugs

Consumption of alcohol, tobacco and similar substances is clearly an issue pertaining to health and wellness, diet, and weight loss. Dietary and intake behaviors and mistakes affect overall body chemistry. For that obvious reason, some discussion about this topic is warranted in this book. It will be from the standpoint of the effects on body chemistry (detail about addiction to them as substances will be provided in other books).

Alcohol is a substance that will have an immediate effect on your organs and your overall chemistry. Complete abstinence from alcohol—whether it's in the form of beer or wine or hard liquor—is best. It is bad for your liver. If you want your body to function at an optimal level, you have to consider the reality that alcoholic beverages are not nutritional substances. They are chemical disruptors. There may be benefits from red wine such as the compound trans-resveratrol, but the toxicity of the wine outweighs such benefits.

Ingesting any type of smoke into the lungs is a huge mistake. The lungs are digestive organs, but only for air and nutrients such as oxygen. The lungs are not designed as filters for the contaminants in tobacco and cannabis.

There are other very significant dangers associated with smoking. They include bringing carbon monoxide into the lungs and the very high level of irritation that heated smoke brings to the inner surfaces of the lungs. Smoking is a disaster.

If you choose to use marijuana because you like its effect, you're far better off ingesting it through the mouth and letting it be filtered through the digestive channels of the stomach and the intestines. The digestive system is a phenomenal filter for toxic substances.

I want to emphasize that you don't need any of these compounds. But if you choose to use them, use them in a safer way.

The ideal way to consume alcohol is in drinking limited amounts of Kombucha: Its alcohol content is low, and there are some probiotics in the drink. But Kombucha should not be used as a primary source of hydration; doing so would constitute overuse. Most Kombucha drinks have refined sugars that are added (primarily to be reliable food for the good bacteria that need to feed and replicate in the liquid), but some are made with honey.

85. What About Coffee?

Think of coffee as one of the few substances to which the aphorism "less is more" applies. I know that it may be difficult to hear these words because we rely very heavily on intoxicating, stimulating substances to get us through the day and help us deal with our emotions and lives.

We tend to minimize how important things such as coffee, alcoholic beverages, and other foods serving as stimulants or depressants are to our sense of control and calmness. Coffee is a very, very powerful plant medicine. It gives us a very subtle feeling of power. It gives us the ability to numb bodily sensations and emotions: Not stopping them completely, but acting as a buffer.

When something works for us we tend to overuse it, thinking that more is better. And we can go for a very long time without seeing any physical consequences. But in the meantime the psyche is affected in a big way. Coffee can turn us into somebody else completely. If you use it too much, it will turn you into someone other than the person you want to become. So you need to pull back from your overuse of it a little bit at a time.

Be very mindful when you drink coffee so that you can be aware of its effect on you; even a very small amount should suffice for that. You must know what effect you are expecting from the coffee.

Are you looking just for the taste, and if so, what's the emotional effect of the taste? If the pleasurable effect of the taste is what you're looking for, you probably need far less of it than you currently drink in order to savor that taste.

Are you caught up in the habit of going to your favorite coffee place, saying hello to the barista, filling your mug, and then feeling as if you've completed a vital task? If that's the case then you need to be aware of the pattern.

I disengaged from a major coffee place by just going there two times, coming in and saying hello, ordering a coffee, paying for it and then leaving it behind. I broke the pattern.

I didn't want to drink their coffee because quite honestly it tasted like diarrhea and it didn't relax me. I felt like I was a drug addict going to the methadone clinic. I wanted to change my behavior.

I came up with the aforementioned silly ritual to interrupt my pattern. Then I just started making cold brew coffee at home. It was so easy.

You can get the effect you want while going through a painless withdrawal. The way to do that is to gradually pull back on all of the rituals surrounding your coffee drinking. You don't want to get emotional grounding from the substance of coffee.

There are other ways to feel grounded that are far more powerful. Here's an example: Start your morning with your eyes closed, find the light in the middle of your forehead when your eyes are closed, and chase it for five minutes. Don't get distracted from practicing this; it's an introduction to meditation. If we are able to get peace of mind from practices such as meditation, eventually we won't need substances to serve as boosters we use in daily life.

Coffee has two types of effects—its physical effects and its effects on the personality. Some of us really feel that we desperately need the edge it gives us. But we're drinking it excessively, not being mindful when we drink it, and we're in denial about the negative effect that it has on our body chemistry.

I recommend that you take a quiet moment to consider this information and think about how you can cut down (or even quit completely). Go as slowly as you need to in order to be successful at cutting down; you need not quit right away. Go at your own pace. Just remember that your progress will be limited by whatever dietary mistakes you engage in.

The way that I phased down coffee was to only drink about 4-5 ounces of black, cold brew coffee with about one ounce of a homemade oat milk. I didn't need any sweetener.

However you decide to drink your coffee, I strongly suggest you eliminate using dairy from a cow immediately (even if it's only an ounce or so). It's completely unnecessary, and it's not good for you. Certainly eliminate any processed or artificial sweeteners.

Please consider the following suggestion for getting the maximum effect from coffee while reducing the amount that you drink (this suggestion works for reducing alcohol consumption as well): Take your time while drinking your cup of coffee. Talk to it directly, telling it what you'd like it to do for your mind and body. I agree that this sounds totally ridiculous. But you have nothing to lose, so please try it.

Set a target date for when you wish to be completely free of it (maybe a couple of months, maybe 10 years, your call) and hold yourself accountable for what you want to do. Certainly if you have a serious illness then it will be much more urgent to quit quickly.

Energy drinks that use caffeine and taurine to the extreme are incredibly unhealthy to both the body and the mind. They're like an atomic bomb on your endocrine system.

If you're using those types of products, you've got to become aware of why you're using them and how they affect your behavior. Then you should develop a plan to stop using them, using techniques such as those this book suggests to improve your health and emotional wellness so that you won't need that artificial stimulation. Engage in your meditation, your prayer, and your writing. Really get into figuring out how to surrender energy drinks.

Another thing: When you are drinking coffee in order to balance your chemistry, you should drink at least 16 ounces of water immediately after drinking your coffee. Also make sure that you drink plenty of water throughout the day, not just immediately after "coffee time."

It's quite clear that quitting caffeine is a very difficult thing to do. But you need to be aware that coffee is a mild slow-acting poison of sorts. That's part of the reason why it is so stimulating to our body: When we drink it, our body secretes adrenaline to try to flush that substance out of the body and restore our chemistry back into homeostasis.

Coffee tastes great if you are a coffee drinker, but it's also a compound that acts on your emotional chemistry.

It could subtly change your mood from being low to being high. Coffee is extremely popular because it helps people keep up with the pace of modern life. We're doing so much these days and doing it so fast that we feel we need a substance to energize us.

The question is, at what cost? It's been proven that a cup of coffee (or caffeine in other forms) can benefit the body. But most of the studies are done with a micro perspective on the subject.

For the most part, people who are battling illnesses shouldn't overstimulate their bodies; doing so could make their problems worse. On the other hand, some who are fighting illnesses could benefit from the boost of caffeine to give them a little bit more stimulation. It depends on a number of factors.

Anyone who quits coffee knows that they feel "down" for a period of time following their decision to quit. In a future book I will discuss both physical and mental effects of stimulants (coffee among other things) and the emotional processes associated with quitting them.

In these modern times we collectively consume coffee to extreme excess, ingesting too much caffeine and theobromine. If we stimulate ourselves too much we are accelerating our aging in the process. Consider the following metaphor: If I have a Ferrari and I drive it as fast as it can go, it will break down faster. This is also true with our bodies.

Having said that, I understand the frantic pace of life in our modern times. There are times that we may need a little boost. Coffee is so enmeshed in our culture and lifestyle that I'm more afraid to say "leave coffee out of your diet" that I am to say "leave animal protein out of your diet."

If you're going to drink coffee, make sure that it consists of USDA Organic coffee beans. Coffee beans, like grapes that are used for wine, are sprayed with a ton of pesticides. If you're going to be consuming coffee over many years, it means that slowly and surely if you're not drinking organic coffee then you're drinking something that's part poison.

It's also important to remove all sweeteners from your coffee. Much as we as people have become intellectually desensitized to information and unusual situations in today's world, our taste buds have become desensitized to coffee's flavor because of our overuse of sweeteners and flavorings.

One can simply drink black coffee in a meditative state, as if using it only for medicinal purposes of stimulation and mood changing, and then eat two dates or two figs. Over time you may not crave the sweetness of the fruits and may just appreciate the black coffee by itself.

Coffee is intoxicating and there should be limits to its use. Coffee is no different than all the other plant medicines that are out of the Garden of Eden. The coffee bean is edible and it can be a medicine or a poison depending on how it's used.

I recommend not having more than 8-10 ounces of brewed coffee, or no more than two ounces of espresso, per day. And I would make an effort to skip one day a week. I think two or three cups constitutes overuse by stimulating your body too much, and doing so only for the psychological benefit of keeping yourself up. Inevitably, a reciprocal amount of crash equal to the amount of spike that you get will be the result.

By the end of the day when you feel tired, just let yourself feel tired and prepare yourself to rest rather than be stimulated. Your body will thank you for it.

86. Cacao (Chocolate) and Maca

Ricoa and things like maca stimulate and move the chemistry faster. That doesn't mean that weight loss will occur. Your heart rate might go up, your organs might go faster, you might secrete more hormones. But there's no free ride in your body chemistry. Remember that if you stimulate you must come down and crash.

The ancient people who understood and first used the plants that contained those substances did not abuse them. They used them for specific things and they generally accompanied their use with ceremonies and rituals. They prepared themselves mentally to bring these substances into their bodies to avoid being overpowered by them.

The purpose of a healthy diet is to try to decrease stimulation and increase nutrient value while decreasing caloric intake. The details may be complex, but that is the goal in a nutshell.

87. Other Hippie Weirdo Products

More than likely you've heard the term "superfoods." Another popular term is "adaptogens."

These are buzzwords that are created to sell products. And the buyer should be cautious. If you purchase expensive weirdo products, it usually just means that the value of your urine goes up.

Everything that is nutritious is a superfood to me. If I were crawling across the desert and hadn't eaten in three days, I would consider an apple a superfood. Or I would consider an olive to be the most important meal of my life at that moment.

Be suspicious of anything called a superfood. Such products are often advertised with boasts and claims that are unsubstantiated or false. For example, a product may be touted as being loaded with protein, but if you study the label you may find that not to be true.

Superfoods sometimes have very few standard macronutrients and micronutrients, such as carbohydrates, fats, proteins, vitamins, and minerals. But they might be very high in substances like flavonoids, antioxidants and phytochemicals. Such compounds can be researched and found to be incredibly valuable for fighting off a variety of diseases and building up the immune system.

I'm very much in favor of those things, as long as the people who sell them take the time to research and get peer-reviewed papers and documented scientific studies. Many people in the supplement industry won't do those things because doing so challenges their products' efficiency and their own economy.

The main thing to understand is that if you have limited processed food, eliminate dairy, and follow the other guidelines of this book, you can become very healthy: You shouldn't need to wash your face with chia from the rainforest while having a coffee enema to make sure that you make it to age 99. I believe that all of the various tricks and cheats enable people to continue unhealthy dietary practices. The tricks and cheats exact significant cost to body chemistry in the long run.

88. USDA Organic Certified Produce

My company Juice Press proudly held a USDA Certification. I know firsthand from dealing with the United States Department of Agriculture (USDA) that their certification process is rigorous. Inspections are conducted by an incorruptible culture of privatized certification companies that would risk a lot if they took shortcuts or if they succumbed to corruption. USDA organic certification requires that not only are your facilities inspected to ensure that all of the processes are up to their standard, but that any kind of chemicals used in the kitchen or an area where products are held must also be approved to meet the high USDA organic standard.

The quality of product from a USDA certified organic food production facility is superb—far better than that of most food products sold in supermarkets. Which begs the question: Why do big supermarkets that pledge to help us and demonstrate deep concerns for the public at large, their workers, the farms, and the environment still use deceptive words to market their products to their customers? Answer: Profit.

If I took you on a tour to show you the best and the worst markets in the USA, I would point out to you how they are all littered with marketing words that fool us into making choices that will negatively impact our chemistry.

You definitely do not want pesticides in your foods. They are poison for killing small creatures and they alter our chemistry too. Either quickly or slowly, they will eventually have a deleterious effect on our genetic material, our cells, the tissues of our body, our organs, and therefore our entire self. All synthetic chemicals ingested into an organic organism will have an intoxicating effect on that organism because they are not pure from this earth.

They are manufactured by man using harmful sciences. Are there helpful man-made chemicals? Yes; just not pesticides. They help farmers to create something unnatural that sickens and kills.

I am assuming that by now there are very few people who live in economically developed countries who would refute that pesticides have a negative effect on the environment. That in itself should be the primary reason to avoid "conventional" produce and products.

Our government subsidizes the wrong types of things. Everything should be grown organically. It's crucial for the health and the well-being of our planet. The costs associated with long-term exposure to the variety of toxins that we take in from the pesticides that are sprayed on products far outweigh savings at the supermarket.

Pesticides seep into the soil and easily leach into the edible fibers of produce: So even if a particular type of produce has a very thick skin, in one way or another you're getting a dosage of poison with your food.

You should not be completely paranoid about this situation, because that unhappiness can make you just as sick. But you should consider making the switch to organics. It's well beyond the scope of my knowledge to talk to you about similar quality standards for livestock raising and other flesh food industries. But if you eat the flesh of an animal, I encourage you to do your best to ensure that the flesh is pure and uncorrupted.

PART 5
ADVANCED WORK INTO ACTION

89. Vital Force

The first rule of the diet is recognizing that your body is a total healing machine. It operates and functions solely on the energy that your diet provides.

A small percentage of energy is generated by your mentality and your psychological functioning, but this is in extremely limited supply. I call it "vital force," and I was told of it by my mentor. Vital force is a very small amount of energy that is directly attached to your immune system. It must be preserved in order to keep the immune system on high alert. We must not rob ourselves of our critical supply of this vital force.

They have no word for this energy supply in scientific circles. It's virtually undetectable. But it is the source that we use up if we are ever completely empty. It's the energy that a person must access when they know they're going to die if they don't find safety, metaphorically or literally. You don't feed this vital force—it's a by-product of clean living and having the right overall lifestyle.

Vital force is the energy left over, after all of our daily energy needs are accounted for. This remaining energy is a direct benefit to the energy needed for our immune system. We drain this supply with stress and with needing to clean up and detox from a diet loaded with excessive amounts of toxins.

What toxins? Anything that we consume that is disruptive to normal chemistry and healthy cellular function is intoxicating to us. Such things include alcohol, drugs, junk food, excessive amounts of protein, and a number of other substances. And overeating in and of itself is intoxicating.

Because you're alive right now and are reading this, vital force is still intact in you. But I'm very hesitant to write out a program or a protocol for creating something that is short-lived and doesn't deliver a person to their own salvation. If you've eliminated processed foods and are not eating too much protein, your dietary needs will become obvious within 24 hours of feeling hunger pains.

90. Getting Rid of Food Contraband

As we progress on our journey to weight loss and a healthy lifestyle, we should always be striving to make it to the next level. This short section describes a very important measure for us to take to help get us there.

People who are extremely determined to quit smoking need to dispose of all of their "contraband"—items that tempt them and enable them to relapse. Such things include ashtrays, lighters, matches, pipes, and cigarette cases. If we as toxic food addicts, compulsive overeaters, or just individuals with difficulty breaking bad dietary habits are deadly serious about overcoming our problems, we too have to surrender our contraband.

The first action is to meet with our spouses, partners, children, office workers, or other significant people in our lives and set a date to clean out all of the cabinets, refrigerators and food storage areas in our main places of eating and living. That means you're going to throw out all of the garbage in every category, including impure processed spices, kosher salt, ice cream, candy, cereals, junky breads, cookies, cakes, pretzels, sodas, food coloring, white sugar, white flour, pastas, canned nonsense, and many other items.

You're doing everyone a long-awaited favor by getting rid of all that garbage. In doing so, we reduce our risk of overeating and eating poorly, and we reduce the risk of disease and suffering that is caused by processed crap. Out of sight, out of mind. We have to get it out of the house. We have to do it! It's such a big move. It's a major step.

Get prepared for this step: It's a tough one. Get a good friend to help you. Once you start, no hoarding. No excuses. Get some big garbage bags and start dumping. Don't donate it to the poor—that's a really shitty thing to do, because no one needs that garbage in their bodies.

Afterwards, go to the biggest health food store in town and stock up on things you need. Stock up on things that go bad, on things with clean ingredients, and—very important—make sure that the items that you select are organic.

Doing so is not just about the pesticides. It's about the quality of the food that passes scrutiny by the USDA. This scrutiny that all certified organic businesses have to be held accountable to is what makes the USDA great. It truly is an excellent quality control standard.

My former business was USDA Organic, and I went through their inspection process annually. It was tough. We had transparency with everything from our farms, to our cleaning supplies, and to the processes in the kitchen. Everything was scrutinized to a very high standard.

So, it bears repeating: Always be sure that you purchase and use foods and products that are certified as being USDA Organic.

91. Late Night Safety Measures to Protect Against Emotional Eating

You must understand your own moods and emotional shifts that occur throughout the day—particularly those that tend to repeat themselves and those that occur during the evening or late at night. Doing so will help you protect yourself from being overwhelmed or "caught off guard" when cravings occur.

We're all slightly different regarding those urges and how we respond to them. Some feel satisfied with a single cup of morning coffee. Others drink it in excess when they feel anxiety. Others like the ritual and habit, and/or the adrenalin spike that coffee provides. The emotional benefits can also include a person's feeling grounded or secure when having a cup. Unfortunately, such positive benefits are far outweighed by the negative effects of emotional or physical addiction to the substance(s). And this is also true regarding junk foods, alcohol, and a myriad of other things.

Anxiety and emotions well up inside of all of us every day. During certain periods, particularly late in the evening, many seek a sweet snack, a cup of coffee, or an alcoholic beverage to give them a distraction, change their chemistry, or feel grounded. But such things are not harmless gestures. They are addictive behaviors. And anyone trying to overcome an addiction of any kind needs to abstain from addictions or addictive behaviors of every kind.

You know your own patterns. You know that when you feel down you'll be most likely to want to reach out for something. You know that when you feel up and victorious you might want to reach out for something to "celebrate." You may want to reach out for something all the time, or just at specific times.

What I have discovered is that most people act out their lowest impulses relating to food after the sun goes down. This is the time when people feel really comfortable about eating late at night to be social. The late night dinners are often accompanied by the warm and soothing feelings of alcohol. We let our guards down and then go for the super rich dessert on the table.

People can do very strange things in the privacy of their kitchens. I know people who wake up in the middle of the night just to open the doors of their refrigerators for feelings of reassurance. Many end up eating after doing that even though they weren't intending to before they opened the doors.

Such behavior patterns are the ones that you must become familiar with. You have to discipline yourself to have replacement behavior patterns during the times you know you're most likely to act out. You must schedule things that bring you comfort and relaxation and do them instead of acting out with bad dietary choices. This is a good time to practice an evening meditation. This is a good time to do some very slow-paced, easy yoga postures that don't stimulate you, maybe while you're watching television.

I do certain things to unwind at the end of the day. I have to have a time of day where I plug in my phone to charge and I turn it upside down. I need a shower at the end of the day to transition from the day to the period of time for rest. I like to do some push-ups and squats at nighttime to tire me out; it doesn't keep me awake and it feels good on my body.

But I have to be cautious around 10 PM, when I'm prone to getting into mischief. That's when I need to remind myself that I'm winding down, that I had a great day, that I'm going to enjoy my sleep, and that I'll start over again tomorrow.

I very strongly recommend that you do some writing work about the times of day during which you feel compulsive. What are your triggers? In what ways do you act out? What benefit do you think that the acting out gives you?

This is important. Don't just read that and tell yourself that the assignment isn't that important or that you don't have time for it. That's just laziness on your part.

Writing out the things that you've thought through regarding your time of day compulsion triggers will cause you to learn things about yourself. It will stimulate you to the degree that you will think of many solutions and alternatives to acting out. Subsequently, you will have well-thought-out plans of action to engage instead of the toxic behaviors that tempt you at those particular times.

This is especially useful if you do it in coordination with other recovery measures. You can pray, meditate, and talk with your therapist or friends and family members about your triggers and what goes on in your overall emotional world during different times of the day. Such feedback is crucial.

92. Set Eating Times for Each Meal. Create Repetition and a Pattern

It's very important to start certain people off with one month of eating large portions of healthy foods, having them eat a lot more calories than necessary: That helps train their minds to think that they are full. In the beginning when some are changing eating patterns, they are not only going into a calorie deficit, but they're also afraid of being hungry. They often feel hungry because the stomach doesn't know what to tell the brain, and vice versa. The focus at first is to change the pattern of what we eat, not the calorie count.

It's advisable for those changing their eating patterns to set timetables for when they allow themselves to consume food. They should set hours such as at 5:50 PM, or 12 noon to 7 PM, or 11 to 6, and then consume no solid food. Then, if hunger ensues, they should consume liquids—anything ranging from water to fresh raw juice. Eventually, the need for fresh juice during those times would go away.

93. Avoiding Fad Diets

Losing weight is not easy. Fad diets may work in the short term. But they will generally disappoint us as we are likely to revert back to old habits at some point.

There is little value in following diet plans that are loaded with high amounts of fats or high amounts of protein. These are short-term tricks played on your chemistry and they will lead to problems. Diets that sell you chemically processed shakes are not the solution either.

They are the wrong diets for our long-term health. In my opinion, the Keto diet, Paleo diet, the Atkins diet, the Zone diet, and so many others waste valuable time and often intoxicate the body in the long run.

Diet plans that do not incorporate psychological and emotional measures are incomplete. This is so because they don't place tools such as talk therapy and step-by-step instructions on how to reorganize your total outlook at your feet. Such diet plans are centered on measures that don't get to the roots of your diet-related problems.

People eat for emotional and psychological reasons, not just for sustenance. Thus, people by choice remain at the body weight they choose on a conscious and subconscious level. I won't prescribe a fad diet to anyone for these and other reasons.

The Keto diet is just completely wrong from a health and longevity perspective. I will not give it special attention in a book on nutrition, because it's not sound human nutrition. No more so than smoking crack or inhaling whippets is nutrition.

My website www.goodsugar.life has support articles, including more disturbing information on the Keto diet. Besides what you read on my website, be cautious about most of the things that you read on the internet. Much of that information is incomplete, just flat out wrong, or biased because of attempts to sell products based on bogus science.

94. Ancient Ayurvedic and Chinese Medicine Diets

I have positive things to say about the Ayurvedic Diet and the Chinese Medicine Diet because they avoid processed food and protect the earth. However, I do not believe in pinpointing a body type down to wet or dry, hot or cold, spicy or not spicy (as these methods propose). I believe many of those assessments are based on anecdotal evidence and abstract, unprovable sciences.

I am not a disbeliever in western science. But I don't like western medicine unless the person taking it is sick and that medicine is vital. And I despise the western food industry, which has a direct link to the western pharmaceutical industry. Both industries are regulated by the United States government, but very little is done regarding educating the public and providing the best products for ensuring good health.

Having said that, Ayurvedic medicine is old and dated science to me. It was developed without laboratories and devices to help prove hypotheses. The field attracts a multitude of quacks as well as some sincere practitioners.

Certain aspects of the Ayurvedic diet are anecdotal. This is the case because usually when a person begins their journey on that type of diet, they're also doing a number of other things that may cause positive results to happen.

Consider this example: Perhaps your doctor tells you that you're under a lot of stress and you've got to change your diet or you're going to have a heart attack. Then you cut out meat from your diet and start riding a stationary bike. You then start taking lots of vitamins, and you try meditation twice a week.

A couple of months go by and you drop a few pounds. And all of a sudden your numbers are back where they're supposed to be and your doctor is blown away by the turnaround. When he asks you what your secret is, you tell him you started riding a bicycle at home.

Seeking to build a fortune, the doctor then writes a book on how to reverse the risk of heart disease through bike riding. But he leaves out all of the other good things that you did or bad things that you quit doing. Leaving out many things, the doctor only wrote about one piece of the puzzle.

So I contend that the primary things that work about the Ayurvedic diet are avoiding processed food and reducing intake of animal protein. Those who practice it likely make a number of lifestyle changes for the better. And many of those things may be part of the puzzle of why their lifestyles in general and their diets in particular have worked well for them.

My opinion makes me less popular in the health food movement. But I've formed my opinion based on study, personal experience, consultation with experts, and formal and informal interviews with people who had very bad experiences with ineffective treatments given by homeopathic scholars.

I could write volumes on ridiculous stories I've heard. My favorite is the treatment that entails placing a homeopathic medicine on the body of a patient to see if the patient's muscular system agrees with the medicine being selected. All that most of those patients really needed were high doses of probiotic supplements to help balance their digestive systems after years of antibiotic treatments.

The needs and fears of patients make them vulnerable to ineffective treatments. I have no doubt that such treatments are often administered by very well-meaning practitioners. And I am all for natural remedies, even if they are not scientifically proven, but only if they help the patient. But the patient needs to discover quickly if more serious intervention is needed, especially if time is of the essence.

I believe in the use of plant medicines of all kinds, and certainly in the efficacy of herbal concoctions when they are administered by brilliant people. I very much appreciate western-trained doctors who have an open mind and keep far eastern books open at the same time.

The most trustworthy doctor is the one whose first prescription is a radical diet and lifestyle change. I respect people in the medical field who are courageous and who speak their minds to their patients. It's always wonderful to hear a western-trained practitioner tell their patients that their biggest hope for improvement lies in changes to their diets, lifestyles, and attitudes.

95. About the Term "Biohack"

The term "biohack" is presently used a lot in connection products sold by some in the supplement or health and wellness industry. It's a marketing term that has nothing to do with reality.

The concept of "biohacking" doesn't exist. Usually, "biohacking" is a term being used by someone who wants to sell you a packaged, processed product.

We're all suckers for good marketing of products that make desirable promises, but the body does not need a hack. The body is a machine that has incredible self-healing powers provided that you use it in accordance with its natural path.

There's no pill that's going to slow down your aging process or get rid of a mother-in-law that you can't stand. But there are a few biohacking processes. One is to eliminate processed food, junk food, and garbage from your diet. That's a biohack if ever there was one.

Another biohack is to stop buying ridiculous products and stop going on intoxicating diets. Some of the products out there now that are considered to be biohacks would be terrible for people with any type of inflammatory illness, diabetes, or cancer.

The real problem is that people want to continue their lifestyle patterns that are very detrimental to their health. Rather than ceasing our bad lifestyle choices, we want something to fix us so that we can go back to making our mistakes.

I know that it's difficult to stop making mistakes regarding dietary and other health-related choices. It's also difficult to overcome food addictions and other compulsive behavior patterns that lead to health problems of many types.

My message has a very limited audience. This is so because I won't sell feeling good at the price of intoxication of the body. What I want to sell you is enlightenment. I want to sell you better health facilitated by your own participation in it. I want to help make you well.

Being well is also a mental process. You can't just fix your physical body and leave your mental health unchecked; the two entities are inextricably connected. The body and the mind interact in ways that not even science can understand yet.

So another biohacking process I can highly recommend is understanding that you must set your mind on improving both your mental and physical health. You must make doing that a daily practice.

Laziness and fear will be impediments to your progress in doing so, so you must put them aside. To ensure that you will progress in improving mental and physical health, seek out a coach and one or more good mentors.

Please get it out of your mind that there is a bone broth out there that's going to solve all of your problems. There's no collagen supplement, there's no vitamin B12 energy supply, there's no multivitamin, there's no probiotic, there's no mineral, there's nothing like that out there that's going to fix all of your problems.

The solution to all of our problems is to go right to the root causes of them. The root causes of our problems stem from our attitudes and thoughts, as well as from our diet and lifestyle patterns. It's time to pick them apart and make whatever corrections are necessary.

Doing so may not be easy, but it can be done. And the rewards that you will get if you choose to do so will be overwhelmingly satisfying.

96. Fasting and Juice Cleanses

Fasting and juice cleanses are not fad diets, and in my opinion their main use should not be weight loss. A juice fast can promote weight loss if you are in a caloric deficit, though, because juice fasts may help you become more efficient biologically and psychologically. These fasts and cleanses are both powerful ways to allow your chemistry to have total control over bodily cleanup for longer periods of time each day.

Fasting is a way to correct chemistry problems, including insulin resistance and inflammation. Most doctors I know hate this statement. I believe that is because of a lack of experience on their part.

Short fasts, say from evening last meal to 12 noon of the following day (15-17 hours), are a great long-term diet pattern change. I highly recommend fasting as frequently as you like, especially if you don't mind a very slight and manageable feeling of hunger.

Juice fasting went through a fad phase because it was what the public seemed interested in for 5-7 years. **However, juice fasting has been practiced for more than 75 years with many proponents and tremendous results across a wide spectrum of people.**

Before that, water fasting was an important part of many cultures' diet and lifestyle patterns.

Juice cleansing is always a viable option to start a new eating pattern and to change the way we feel about vegetables and fruits altogether. Eventually, if we are to return to our primal health, we will have to incorporate and rely primarily on plants for our sustenance.

Please Note: Juice cleansing and fasting in the context that I am discussing here is extraordinarily safe. It's certainly far less dangerous than the standard American diet, such as that diet is and as it is taught and followed at this point in time. Having said that, if a person has any form of anorexia or Body Dysmorphic Disorder (BDD), a diet with this type of control may be triggering and may set that person off on a long cycle of negative diet patterns.

It's necessary to identify the intentions that you have regarding diet and fasting practices. If your intention is either overtly or secretly just to lose weight, be skinny and get rid of fat, the methods and practices that I'm describing cannot work. Abstractly speaking, your body will not cooperate if you do not have the right intentions behind these types of healing preparations and practices.

A healthy intention for fasting is doing it for the purposes of cleansing and detoxifying various systems of the body. In addition to cleansing and detoxifying systems, fasting can also focus on things such as helping the body to cleanse the blood and facilitating cleansing of the lymphatic system.

The body should be able to do all such things on its own. However, we impede the body's natural healing mechanisms because of our unhealthy diets and lifestyles. By taking a break and not making dietary mistakes, we let the body optimize its cleansing functions at least for that period of time.

If we integrate emotional healing, good behavior practices, positive attitude exercises, juice fasting, and a sustainable long-term healthy diet, that is what's considered to be a holistic program. I believe that many doctors and people in the medical industry are afraid of this concept; perhaps they are fearful that somehow they will be left out if such holistic programs become very popular.

I know that not every doctor thinks that way, but perhaps many do on a subconscious level. The doctor by trade needs a person to treat. A doctor-patient relationship could become unintentionally corrupted if the patient heals from methods outside of that doctor's purview.

Doctors and other healthcare practitioners have to remind themselves that above all else their deep hope is that their patients heal. Hence, doctors and other healthcare professionals have to have **extremely** open minds. They must learn a great deal more than what they are traditionally taught.

They must experience it as well. I served juice fasts to scores of PhDs and MDs. The ones that I tracked loved doing them. Although there's some controversy surrounding simple juice fasts, there should not be. There are many published peer-reviewed papers on water fasting. Yoshinori Ohsumi, a Japanese cellular biologist, was awarded the Nobel Prize in Medicine in 2016 for his research on how cells recycle and renew themselves. Fasting activates autophagy, which helps slow down the aging process and has a positive impact on cell renewal.

On their website, The University of Southern California states, **"Fasting for 72 hours can reset your entire immune system."**

There might not be indisputable scientific data on juice cleansing. My hypothesis is that if a water fast is effective and safe, then a similar duration juice fast is also effective to a smaller degree. It is also easier and safer: This is the case because all of the nutrients in juice are left in with the produce's water. Your body will have fuel, as well as most, if not all, of the nutrients it needs for healing and immunity.

The duration that you might attempt to do a water fast is really based on your overall health conditions. I do not recommend that anyone should jump into a water fast without consulting their doctor about it. This should especially be the case with individuals who take medications.

I served hundreds of thousands of people at Juice Press. I watched tens of thousands jump into juice cleanse durations of between three and 45 days. I never saw one negative side effect occur. I never heard of, nor was I presented with information about, a single situation where an individual was put into danger because of juice fasting. Not only were there no problems, but there were countless success stories. I witnessed so many positive transformations that I was often tearful from joy.

I suggest that you make all of the conditions right for a juice fast and then follow a protocol that is reasonable. I don't recommend that people do long-term juice fasts without supervision from an expert. Some people may experience emotional problems when being deprived of their regular behavior and diet patterns: Certainly, they would need considerable support under such conditions. So, I encourage juice fasting, but recommend that those who choose to do it should proceed with caution.

97. Intermittent Fasting: Create Longer Periods of Daily Abstinence Before Eating

Shortening the daily window that you consume food is a way to allow your chemistry to have a longer duration of time and control to clean up your body. This is called intermittent fasting, and it is not a fad. I don't think the word "fasting" is appropriately used for this particular practice; you wouldn't say, "I am on a fast" when abstaining from food in between breakfast and lunch.

Intermittent fasting is a sustainable and healthy pattern to follow for almost all types of people. I am certain there are people who would not do well with not eating at regular more common intervals.

It bears mention that while sleeping you are experiencing the benefits of abstinence. When you are asleep, besides resting the limbs and muscles, you are resting the brain. In this rested state, the energy you expend is cleaning up your entire body chemistry.

I mentioned this before, and I'll mention it again, giving a little more detail this time.

••

My highly recommended tip: If you want to continue consuming exactly what you are consuming now, in terms of both calories and content, change one pattern—never eat after sunset.

••

In the summer months you can eat later than in the winter months. The time to refrain from solid food is determined by the time the sun sets; for example, around 5:00 PM during the winter months and around 7:30 PM in the summer months. **If you want to lose weight in a healthy manner, decide that you will eat NO SOLID FOOD after dark.**

For the first six months, have green juices at night if you are hungry. Drink water throughout the night. **No solid food**. If you consume alcohol you must cut it off by sunset to put this tip into practice.

In this pattern change you are following the body's natural circadian rhythm, which is on a 24-hour clock—work, rest, work, rest. When the sun goes down, the optic nerves signal the hypothalamus gland that it's time to clean house. Not work.

Without a filled stomach, you take control over your entire chemistry. You give your body free reign to do its healing magic. Try this program with the consent of your doctor, priest, rabbi, or whoever you feel medically or spiritually accountable to. You will see dramatic positive improvements.

I want to be clear that if you don't find it reasonable to stop eating after sunset, this does not automatically mean that you will be unhealthy. It's just that not eating after sunset is strongly encouraged because the positive effects are profound.

98. Details Regarding Fasting Practices

Healthy fasting, not deliberate deprivation to shed unwanted body fat, is without a doubt a vital tool in the broad view of lifestyle and diet patterns. People with serious illnesses who have the proper supervision (very important!) can have miraculous recoveries following a healthy fasting protocol.

We should not attempt to speed up or slow down our metabolism to lose weight. You cannot slow down your metabolism by eating less; your metabolism is regulated by many things in addition to how many meals you eat in one day.

If we speed our metabolism above where it naturally belongs, the consequence could be that we are aging ourselves or tiring ourselves out faster as well. Let your metabolism be what it is unless your doctor or health care professional has indicated that something is wrong in your body chemistry.

When we feel hunger pains from just being away from food for a few extra hours, it is likely gas pressure releasing or wanting to release, rather than hunger pangs.

99. My Experience With Cravings

I am fascinated by how I lose inches off my waist and become lean within three days of eating only between the hours 11:00 AM and 6:00 PM. By 9:00 AM I am usually hungry. I drink water, and sometimes I have a few sips of a fresh green juice if I can't handle the feeling of hunger.

At times I get fooled by my senses. Sometimes I feel hungry when my body has a need other than sustenance.

I may need a bathroom break, I may be thirsty, I may feel stressed, or I may be having a delayed emotional reaction to something that occurred. Or I may just need to take several deep breaths because my shallow breathing may have created a negative chemistry.

I now take the time to decide what I am feeling before I eat. I determine if my hunger is legitimate, or if instead my body and mind are signalling a different need. This pause in reacting enables me to make the right decision and then take the next right action.

Just by drinking something, my mental cravings subside. I wake up in the middle of the night almost every time when I am doing this type of diet, with memories that were long forgotten. I go back to sleep.

I wake up in the morning, clear and with a feeling of being lighter. I am hungry. I have cravings. I have to do breathing exercises to hang in there. When I take a morning shower and have a plan of action, I can hold out for a long time.

By 11:00 AM I feel ravenous and excited to have a smoothie or some fruit. Both are easy to digest good sugars and important for energy.

The pattern I've described above is a secret weapon in weight loss. But it should be regarded as a healing tool, rather than just as a weight loss technique.

100. Exercise More and More, Get It In

The essential concept of exercise is this: In order to be healthy in both your mind and body, you need to have a balance of movement and rest. Whatever type of exercise you intend to do, the following things are critical: incorporating flexibility, strength, agility, muscular and respiratory endurance, balance, timing, speed, coordination, adaptivity to new physical challenges, complexity of task, willingness to take reasonable risks with your body, and playfulness with the body. Push your body throughout your life to its appropriate limits: If all one can do is lift a single finger one inch off of their bed, they're still conscious and they're still in the game.

Exercise is crucial for both mental and physical health, including weight loss. But I don't have a breakthrough exercise program that will help you lose 19 pounds in two weeks.

Once I lost 14 pounds in 48 hours by skipping rope in a plastic suit and then spending over four hours in a sauna. I did this in order to make a fighting weight in a thai boxing competition; I went from 154 to 140.

It was gruesome. Luckily after I weighed in I had about 12 hours to recover. I weighed in on a Friday at 140 pounds. After I participated in the fight I did some binge eating to compensate for my exhaustion and deprivation. On Sunday, after my fight and my binge eating, I got on the scale to see what I had done to myself. My weight was 168 pounds. I ate so much after my fight because of the deprivation I had put myself through for two months that I managed to gain 28 pounds in two days.

Much of the weight I had lost was just straightforward water. I had sucked myself dry of water by using old-school fighter techniques taught to me by my trainers. So it wasn't surprising that when I started to hydrate again I put on that much more weight in water. It was horrible.

There are far more sustainable exercise and diet programs. The most sustainable lifestyle program is to think of your weight loss as something that you're going to master over the course of 12 months. It would involve the typical amount of weight loss that a person could handle over a longer period of time. It would also include all of the patterns a person would have to change to ensure that they'd become routines.

It's necessary to build on your successes little by little, be forgiving and patient with yourself, and not push yourself for an overnight result. The desire for an overnight result is the nature of the thinking of an addict.

We unfortunately have desires for immediate gratification. And sometimes we act out addictively to suffocate the lack of the ability to deal with the frustration of not getting what we want right away.

You can retrain yourself to stop doing that just by being mindful of it and taking action to stop. If you're not a self-starter, then you have to do a lot of writing and also have a good therapist to discuss these issues with.

Some people would say that you have to get to the root cause of every single maladaptive behavior, but that might take a lifetime. You do have to get to the behavior causes eventually, but in the meantime if you're strong enough you can take action and create new behavior patterns.

The question is, what is it that's going to motivate you to take necessary steps? What's going to motivate you to get into your new program for the first week? The first day is the hardest day, because that's when the fear is throbbing in our minds.

Human beings usually don't like to change in this way because it requires discomfort. But the only discomfort you'll feel will be some aches and pains from great workouts (and possibly some hunger pains).

Exercise will be phenomenal for you once you get into the pattern of doing it. The idea is to drive yourself to feel the deep desire of wanting to move every day in some way that you know will be beneficial to you.

•••

Human beings are designed to get into action and move. Our bodies were designed to endure a lot of movement. We're not meant to be sedentary creatures.

•••

For a machine as complicated as an airplane or a human being not to break down, the parts were designed to stay in motion somehow. An airplane has some downtime, and gets mechanical maintenance. Human beings rest and go to sleep, and their bodies have biological mechanical processes for maintenance during those times.

The right amount of physical exercise keeps the muscles strong, the bones dense, the hormones flowing, the sweat dripping, the removal of body toxins happening, and the emotional chemistry being in a state where it needs to be.

A body in motion stays in motion. That's applicable to planetary objects and to the human body as well. If you keep yourself moving with the right amount of exercise, combined with the right amount of rest and a wholesome diet, you will do very well.

Throughout the book I mention yoga very lightly and in passing. I want to really put it in your mind that yoga is a comprehensive system of physical and emotional wellness. Understanding what this yoga thing is all about takes time and practice. First, yoga is a great way to exercise and challenge the body in a complete way.

The philosophies of yoga are not religious in nature or contentious with your primary religious beliefs. Yoga philosophy is complementary. You can work out a lot of issues by enjoying the pure teachings of the ancient far east. I find the studies to be intellectually stimulating and they put me into action in the best way possible—mindfully.

No other practice has given me this relationship to my body and mind, my breathing and my emotions. I practice something every day. No days off. Two days a week, my practice is so minimal that it's what you would call a day off, but I am still keeping basic routines and patterns. I cannot afford to take a day off from my healthy patterns. The time off leads to forgetting. It's that simple for a person like me. I need daily routines.

There are other comprehensive systems similar to yoga such as Tai Chi, but I found yoga is more suitable for my "taste buds." The purpose of well-practiced yoga is to tire the body to make relaxation easier. Once we are relaxed, the purpose of yoga is to control breathing and practice controlling the thoughts and distractions in our mind.

When we begin to achieve the ability to focus on a singular thought or object, the quiet in the mind allows us to receive a new mental signal from somewhere deep inside. This description is only a teaser. Yoga exercise and meditation are paired as a complete practice. You are practicing yoga right now if you pull in your abs, tighten your thighs and become aware of your breathing.

101. The Mindset of Exercise

Everyone has a different comfort level regarding how much exercise they can handle. But if you observe children, you'll note that they are lazy to do anything that doesn't feel fun and playful. If you hate exercise, you've got to retrain yourself; you'll have to find a lot of inner strength to start from ground zero. But I highly recommend that whatever physical exercise you start with, make sure that it's fun. You'll be more motivated to play and have fun instead of doing something that feels hard, painful, or boring.

Exercise should be spontaneous—not always programmed (unless you're training for something). I think it's really helpful to mix up your exercise. One day play tennis, the next day practice yoga, the next day try something new that you've never done before, like stand up paddle boarding. I think it's really important to have your regimens and routines, provided they don't stop you from learning new things and seeking adventure and fun. Depending on where you're at with your body, strenuous activity may feel like torture for you. But you have to believe that with repetition, your outlook on this will likely change. It's hard to believe that something you have been doing in your exercise routine can eventually become a habit you look forward to if you keep at it.

After you overcome that initial obstacle of laziness, you've got to look into whether or not you're fearful of using your body. Some people are afraid to get physical because they don't want to be sore or they don't want to get hurt. Or they just don't know what they're afraid of but they're afraid of something, because they don't like change.

If that describes you, you have some work that you have to do on your own. I have a technique that I found to be very useful regarding this. Whenever I had something pending that I really didn't want to do but it had to get done, I would write out what I had to do in my journal and then pray for strength to get it done. If you asked me who I was praying to in the years that I would work like that, I couldn't have told you. But the act of prayer simply worked to get me motivated most of the time (but not always).

The scientific community knows that a person needs to exert a lot of energy towards their exercise programs. No matter what age a person is, the right amount of exercise is that at which it is somewhat difficult. There are exceptions to the rule, depending on a person's profession or crucial circumstances at a given time. For example, a 23-year-old lunatic professional fighter might train a grueling six hours a day. That much training would kill the average person, but that's what that 23-year-old needs to do. But for a 93-year-old person who's had a stroke, walking down a hallway using a walker might be the appropriate type and amount of exercise.

Set up an exercise program in your daily life that makes you exert a lot of force and makes you feel tired. Don't do this motivated by the way it'll make your abs look chiseled in the sunlight. Do this because of how it affects your mind, your thinking patterns, and your emotional world. It will build your sense of self-esteem, it will set off the right type of hormones that will ensure mood stability, and it will improve the state of your heart and lungs. And it will help you lose weight, provided that you do it in conjunction with the other measures that this book speaks of.

102. Suggested Exercise Types

Exercises as complete as good yoga programs are a way to ensure that you get a chance to move all of your body parts—from your toes, to your spine, to your neck, to your hips, your knees, and your fingers. Yoga is a very complete system of exercise to practice.

I am also a huge fan of walking and running, and depending on your overall health level, weight resistance training as part of a weekly program can be beneficial.

Pilates is a very specific regimen that can make your body very strong and toned and I include it into my variations throughout the year.

There are so many different complete systems available, including Tai Chi, Jiu Jitsu, and American boxing. You should choose something that is fun to you and is something that you will stick with. It may be enough for you to get on the treadmill and run for 45 minutes and then do a 15-minute weight routine. Or you may be a person who loves to cycle, swim, or surf; it's all good. Just move and do it.

You may be an older person, and/or your weight may limit your activities. If this is the case, there's still much that you can do. Walking, stair climbing, sit-ups by the bedside, or doing squats while watching the news are a few options. Just don't let your limitations be an excuse to let yourself become sedentary.

103. Walking Is the Most Important Exercise

When we participate in exercise, we are simply moving. I personally think that "moving" would be a more correct term for referring to the activity of exercise. The body has specific laws and mechanical processes that it must follow, and the most basic law of the body is that if it stays in motion, it will continue to function properly. The most important movement for the body is that of walking.

Walking isn't particularly interesting to young people, who have tremendous energy and want to continually be doing something exciting. There's nothing particularly wrong with that mindset for those who are very young. But many people consider walking to be extremely boring. That really should not be the case—because walking is what our bodies were intended to do. We are migrating creatures by design. And we didn't migrate to our intended destinations by jogging, climbing, swimming, or flying. We migrated to the places where we wanted or needed to be by using our legs.

When you walk at a satisfactory pace, you are triggering and stimulating your neurological system. If you concentrate on positive things while doing so, you are in effect washing your system with good energy. Your entire system benefits in many ways when you walk at a good pace.

While walking, you get cardiovascular exercise. Your balance improves. When you walk and master your posture, you can focus on your breath and your footsteps. You can push away all distractions in the process.

Walking really is crucial. If you don't do it, it's difficult to participate in the process of healing yourself mentally, physically, and psychologically. If you make walking a habit and a ritual, you will experience some degree of relief from any and all psychological problems and anxieties that you're going through at any given time.

Resistance training, yoga, running, climbing stairs, and swimming are all fabulous exercises. By all means, participate aggressively in those things if they are your exercises of choice. But do not neglect walking regularly under any circumstances. Walking has benefits that each and every one of us needs and that cannot be met in quite the same way through any other physical activity.

PART 6

ESSENTIAL MINDFULNESS, MEDITATION, PRAYER, AND SERVICE

104. Relax Before Meals and Focus During Mealtimes

This is the least complex of the various steps I've listed in this book, yet it's extremely important (as are all the others). At first glance, this simple step may seem to be somewhat in contrast to statements made in other parts of this guide. But it isn't, and I'll explain why.

There are certain things that most people do every day of their lives that are lacking in any kind of structure—specific periods of time set aside for freedom, exploration, or "play" of some sort. Some might consider such times as being a bit wasteful. But that is absolutely not the case (unless of course those periods of freedom, play, and time are abused by overuse and other factors).

Before meals, some enjoyable but unstructured time is very helpful for the purpose of freeing the mind from stress. This time could be spent taking a walk, sitting on your patio, lying on a beach looking at the ocean, or doing one of an infinite number of other things. But it's imperative that this time should not be spent thinking about problems, planning, checking emails, or doing anything else that requires focused thought.

After spending your unfocused time, you should then shift to a time of being focused—specifically, being focused on the meal that you will then eat. You should think of nothing else but your meal.

Serve your food to yourself and your family on beautiful plates, beautiful glasses, and/or beautiful bowls. Then, as you eat, think of the elements in the food that is nourishing your body.

Think of where the food came from. Think of how the food will improve your health. Be grateful for the provision of the food, and think of your connection with it.

This is quite contrary to eating patterns in our modern times, and particularly in western culture. We eat fast food for convenience. We have "working lunches" when we are in the midst of time-sensitive projects. We conduct company meetings and training sessions during meals. At times such things are necessary because of circumstances that are largely out of our control. But quite often, that's not the case.

•••

In most things in life, it's extremely important to "be in the moment": To be present for the purpose of doing whatever it is that you are involved in, and to do so without being hindered by distractions, thoughts, and interruptions.

•••

And contrary to popular belief, this is very much the case during mealtimes. As most of us eat three times per day, it makes perfect sense that those times should be cherished and used wisely.

105. Visualize Your Body as You Want It to Be

If you're the type of person that tends to read books like this very slowly and pick up things over a long period of time, this section might help you gain a deeper focus on the material. This section describes the practice of visualizing success, and it is applicable to many life goals, diet-related and otherwise.

I learned to visualize success in 2004 at 11:30 at night, while backstage warming up to go out in front of a few thousand people and get into a ring to fight. I had trained for three months for this fight, and the crucial moment was coming. I was nervous, not scared, and I had butterflies. After two or three hours of being in the backstage area I was obsessing, and the obsession was weakening my body.

I was distracted by projecting into the future rather than being right there in the moment. I let the future take control over my mind and I made the future more important than the moment that I was in. The only way I could relax myself was to just lay down on the floor in the locker room, using my gym bag as a pillow. I was doing deep breathing exercises, because doing them was the only thing that prevented me from hyperventilating and feeling a sense of panic.

I laid there quietly for an hour and a half with my headphones on, listening to happy music. If I listened to any music that had negative lyrics, my anxiety came back. If I listened to music that was selfish or egotistical, my heart rate increased. But when I dialed in to the right kind of music, it helped me to feel relaxed.

I spent a good hour visualizing myself going into the ring, being confident, being focused, being present, and taking everything moment by moment. I had to visualize myself at the end of the fight holding up my hand and declaring victory. With every fiber of my being, I kept saying to my body, "I'm prepared for this fight and I'm going to win. I'm going to win, I'm going to win."

Later that evening when I was standing in the ring it was surreal. I had to keep myself present and focused. I had to have a little bit of a smile on my face. I didn't want to look fearful. I had to block out the crowd. I had to look at my opponent's face. I kept telling myself seconds before the bell rang, "I prepared for this fight. I'm in great shape. I belong here. I'm going to win!"

I spoke to many great athletes over the years to confirm that they, too, engage in these mental practices to ensure a victory. It's a very effective system that convinces your body that you're okay and that you're going to win. It's important to see yourself victorious, for even just a brief moment, in order to manifest that victory. **You've got to see the win.**

This very powerful technique not only assists athletes in major sporting events, but it will also assist you as you fight your battle for weight loss and weight control. Lay out a towel, lie on your back, and apply the visualization exercise I just described to your own weight loss efforts.

Visualize yourself in the body you want to be in. See it. Work on this for two or three minutes or more every single day. No days off! And while you're at it in this visualization, feel free to see yourself as happy and rich, cruising on your new yacht with a toned stomach. Visualize anything positive that you want. But, all levity aside, this is a very, very important action. As you take this action, make sure that the body that you want to be in is your primary visualization.

106. Meditation: An Introduction

It is with our minds that we moved our way into suffering early in our lives. And it is with our minds that we must unravel the suffering in order to find peace.

A person seeking to do the deep work of emotional healing required for long-term weight loss must practice meditation. It's a requirement to do so to at least some degree.

The length of time for a single session of meditation will vary from one person to another. Some people might only need short periods of time of stillness and focus. But people who are sensitive and particularly prone to addictive behaviors should not miss a day.

Participating in meditation sessions seven days a week is strongly recommended for everyone. This is so because a lot can happen in one day, and the events that occur daily can be incredibly distracting. Subsequently, thinking about things in an unfocused manner can get a person off the path to good health in general and the disciplines necessary for weight control in particular.

Meditation is not a spiritual exercise. You're not trying to make contact with spiritual beings of any kind—that is a separate practice outside of the scope of this work. The meditation practice I'm speaking of entails working to quiet your mind, working towards your becoming an observer.

We must believe that meditation is such an integral part of a self-help regimen that it's probably impossible to attain our goal without it. So, to begin with, what we need to do is just simply find one or two minutes a day to sit quietly. Perhaps you can do so for 10 minutes or longer. But begin the discipline of meditation as you pursue weight loss and a healthy lifestyle. Begin today and continue with the practice. It's an absolute must.

107. For the Most Distracted People in the World

I created this section for those of my friends who are the most distracted people in the world. Some have wives and children. Some have big businesses. They all have their fair share of stress, and then some. Each event that takes place is a distraction from their inner world and from the sense of balance and peace that they want and need. But they're still amazing people with admirable qualities and enviable lives.

The ones I am speaking of are so distracted that they have some difficulty with looking inside themselves. The concept of staying present for a book as loaded with content as this one is too much. And that's OK.

If you're similar to such people but are trying to make improvements to your diet and health, you will make progress if you keep this book close at hand and keep reading it. Pick it up, read any section, put it down, and then ask yourself what you can remember. Read a section twice if it did not sink in the first time.

Find a quiet place away from the demands of your life. Then read; read two sentences if that's all that you can handle. Find a section with an instruction that you can relate to, and then start doing the action that is suggested.

Many people struggle with just starting to journal. Some may avoid it because they subconsciously struggle with facing up to their emotions. Others have difficulty finding time to even write down a few words. Still others have lives that are so glamorous that they're not motivated to do something as apparently mundane and boring as writing.

Just learning to sit and meditate for five minutes could take a lifetime for some people, especially those caught up in big business who are jammed up with massive responsibilities. I helped a CEO friend of mine hide in his boardroom for three days per week, sit on the floor with his back against the wall, and meditate for three to five minutes. It was torture for him. He couldn't sit with himself: He said that he was either so bored or so distracted that it felt like physical pain.

But slowly, little by little, he disciplined himself so that he could use his train ride from Long Island as a time to practice his meditation and hone his focus. He reported to me later that during a four-month period he developed a new feeling of balance and had found his center. If he continues with his efforts he will accomplish his goals.

You can overcome the barriers to emotional healing, peace of mind, and healthy lifestyle pursuit that your distractions pose. Nothing is so imposing that it will prevent you from doing so. But you must work at it. Break down the suggested self-improvement steps that you need to take into smaller steps, and then begin to take each of those steps one by one.

108. Don't Forget Prayer, Even if You're an Atheist

This is not a theological book. I am qualified to talk about prayer in the realm of addiction and recovery, and that is the main context in which I have used prayer before. Outside of the recovery realm, I used prayer when the door of the skydiving airplane would open and it was time for me to jump out. I love the expression "there are no atheists in foxholes."

I surmise that if I pray for my survival and the survival of my friends, then even if I don't have a specific god in front of me, I still believe in something. Or perhaps I'm superstitious. But ever since age 14 I've found prayer helpful at times when I've hit bottom with behaviors that frightened me and made me feel pitiful.

I prayed in the bathroom when I came to the end of a difficult relationship. I prayed for the next best thing to do. It gave me relief. I pray on a frequent basis on my hands and knees that I will stay clean and sober and free from any addictions that would block my consciousness.

I love being open. In my early days of recovery, I got on my knees with my hands clasped together and I begged God to help me, to let me see the lessons in front of me without having to cause any more damage or trauma. I've said the serenity prayer thousands of times in my life. I've even chanted 108 times in a row to try to understand it. I can see for me that just the action of surrendering, without even knowing what I was surrendering to, was immediately lifting.

Many times in my life, this active surrender was the first step of a new beginning. Prayer is the one thing I never overanalyze. I analyze the living daylights out of everything else. But I made a promise to myself a number of years ago that I wasn't going to try to explain God or explain prayer, because I would have considered it to be foolish for me to try.

I have ideas on what God is. It's going to take me about another 387 years to get some of the pieces of the puzzle together and maybe get them in some semblance of order. With that understanding, I will not find myself in a position of preaching about the nature of God. I can talk about creation, the complexity of the human mind, society, my thoughts on the universe, who I think I am, and who I think you are, but I will not try to explain God.

I think that is the right approach for me. I don't want to be distracted by words and explanations. I want to avoid superstition and I want to avoid carrying extra weight. And I want to avoid being afraid of something that is supposed to bring love into my life. So I'm 100% happy to look at the morality in my life and see if I'm up to par with all of the great religions, and that's how I alone will judge myself. I've learned to block out everyone else's judgment of what I do. It took me a very long time to get to that point.

Whatever you choose to call your higher power or God, I recommend very highly that you keep your judgment of your soul between yourself and that God. I wouldn't trust that with anyone on the earth but yourself, and with any entity but God. Will you take away all the judgments and the feelings of guilt and shame? They could be attached to something as wonderful as a deep religious and spiritual worldview. Dwelling on guilt and shame may cause you tremendous stress and anxiety. It could make you want to act out and overeat, or to succumb to another addiction to numb the pain.

All you have to do to pray, my friend, is pick a body position, pick a comfortable place, and start talking. If you're into drama, I recommend you lay flat on your belly with your legs splayed out and your arms stretched out in front of you and then look up at the sky and beg for help if you need it. But if that's too dramatic, then just go watch the sunset and say, "Thank you."

Find whatever ritual works for you and then stick to it. And once you start it, I recommend that you don't make it optional. Do it every day. Do it for five seconds, do it for five hours, whatever suits you. But I recommend that you pray. Get it all out. Say everything you need to say.

It's really wonderful when you're facing the ocean, and it's amazing when you can see a starlit sky and look up at it and whisper some prayers that ascend into it. You can be a proud atheist if you want—that's how easygoing I am.

But there's something to pray for. And it's really worth making it a part of your pattern. In fact, if you're an atheist come up with a whole new set of atheist prayers.

Amen.

109. Positive and Negative Thoughts

The way that addiction works is that there is a union between the body and the mind. The mind tells the body what it wants, and then the body gears itself up for whatever effort it takes to get what it wants. If you're telling yourself that you want to eat compulsively and that you love unhealthy foods, you're sending a confusing signal to your body.

Your body will physically crave those unhealthy foods to reduce the amount of stress caused by any resistance between body and mind communication. So a very important step in addiction recovery is to tell yourself every day with your meditation that you do not want to eat that way any longer: It does not serve you, it does not serve your body, and it does not serve your consciousness.

It's an exercise that I would practice while driving, running, sitting in meditation, during yoga, or during any activity where you can be completely focused on the breath. The breath will carry the thought to the physical body. The breath is like an intermediary; it's both physical and mental. Metaphorically, the breath is like a spirit—it can move back and forth between the physical body and your mental faculties. So it's important that you are consciously breathing when you want to communicate well between the mind and body.

At that point you can think positive thoughts. Be very specific: "I don't need coffee. I don't need caffeine. I don't want to use it anymore. I want to stop it because it holds me back. It makes me feel like a slave to that substance. I want to be liberated from that attachment and others."

Next, go through every unhealthy food or food group and repeat words like that. For example: "I don't want to eat unhealthy things. I don't want to eat cookies. I don't want to eat ice cream. I don't want to eat candy bars. I don't want to eat processed food. I really want to stop eating those things."

It's going to take some time and practice to continually do this to get to the point where it has a dramatic effect. Some don't believe in the process and won't attempt it. Such people don't realize that what they're fighting against is the faulty programming in their minds. They don't realize that quitting unhealthy things is in conflict with aspects of the self and aspects of the mind.

In order to be empowered, you have to integrate the body, the mind, and all thoughts. They should all be in alignment. There's a team inside of your body—the players are the body, the mind, the thoughts, and the super consciousness. You are the coach of the team. You've got to get the players in unison with each other.

Tell yourself these things: "I do not want to be afraid of dying. I do not want to be fearful of anything. I want to open my mind. I want to be a better person." These are the types of messages we have to repeat to ourselves over and over and over again to overwrite the negative messages that play in your mind throughout the day. Those negative messages are on autopilot. They were usually received by way of someone else's messages to us; perhaps it was our parents, our siblings, or our society. There's a broken record playing the same negative songs, and the body resigned itself to these messages.

Some won't believe what I and others say regarding this unfortunate pattern and how to overcome it. It seems metaphysical and esoteric in this day and age that we live in, but it's really just simple physics. The body and the mind are connected in ways that we don't have good explanations for. But many just can't fathom the concept that the body, a physical and visible thing, can connect to the invisible mind.

What they don't realize is that the mind is made of things, as is the body. Thoughts are chemical in nature. Thoughts are actually made up of chemical substances, and the chemicals react and have constant interaction with the entire chemistry of the body. So when you think something that you believe is a negative thought, there's a charge to that thought, and it's a negative charge. The thought will have an impact on your chemistry by doing all the things that something negative in your chemistry would do.

They'll be a reduction of energy. There could be a tightening of the muscles. There can be shortness of breath. All these things bring the physical energy down even lower than it was at the start of the internal dialogue. And when the body is in that lower state, it communicates to the mind, and then the thoughts get pulled down as if through a drain.

Positive thoughts work in the opposite way. When you deliberately think positive thoughts, you're shifting your physical chemistry in a positive way without exhausting yourself. Thoughts such as this will have that effect: "Today I love how the day is going. Look at the beautiful flowers along the highway! It's hot outside and I feel hopeful. I love the way my car runs. I love looking at the foliage on the highway. I'm glad to be alive."

Practices saying these things to yourself in moments that you find yourself becoming bored or disinterested. When you do so, you are building up your resistance to negativity. You will become much more effective at combating negative thoughts that might arise later on.

This will be of tremendous benefit to you—so fill your mind with positive thoughts as often as possible.

110. Gratitude

Gratitude definition: Thankfulness, appreciation, recognition, readiness to show appreciation for and to return kindness.

There's no other state of mind that I can think of that is as beneficial to your chemistry as that of being grateful. There are two ways that I know of that will get you there. One is just a natural response to excitement, elation, pleasure, accomplishment, or any other positive experience. The other is by being contemplative about the situations and the events of our lives.

It doesn't make a difference whether or not you're trying to overcome an addiction or an affliction of some kind. It's a mature practice to find time throughout each day, seven days a week, no days off, to be pensive about the things in our lives that we are grateful for. At certain points in my life I would have had no idea how to relate to those words or put them into action.

When we are very young and have a lot of negative things going on in our lives, the negativity has free reign over our mentality and it drags us down. It's very difficult for young people to just simply make up their minds to change their attitudes about life for the better. This is so because of the great amounts of pain that they feel.

So, young people who are struggling and feel powerless will have a hard time understanding the concept of focusing attention to the positive things in their lives. Doing so is something that should become a lifelong habit. It takes tenacity and practice to achieve the ability to change the course of your mind's natural negative tendencies. Shifting your mind's focus from what's wrong to what's right should be done on a day-to-day, moment-by-moment basis.

So, it takes practice, and it requires a fervent desire to make this shift. And you must also have insight. The insight that's required is knowing either intuitively or by experience that shifting focus is both extremely helpful and not very difficult.

"Having an attitude of gratitude" seems like a platitude to some. It's become a cliché. But think about why clichés become clichés: That happens because their words communicate very powerful, actionable truths that create positive change when they are used as intended. Bottom line: Having an attitude of gratitude is extremely effective in helping you to both achieve better health and to overcome any problems that you experience in life.

I doubt that any one person can tell you exactly how to turn your thinking around from negative thinking to examining your blessings. The way that I learned to do it came much later for me in my recovery—much later than I would have expected and much later than I would have liked.

Shifting to gratitude doesn't mean that you go into denial about certain problems that you have to address. If you're worried about your finances and you think that the solution is just to get grateful, that might lead to a problem: Please don't take what I'm saying here to mean that you should develop the ability to deny reality. What I'm saying is actually just the opposite, and I'll explain why.

Shifting your focus to a grateful state of mind is actually shifting your mind to another reality that's happening simultaneously with some of the more difficult realities. It's not denial of reality—it's an acceptance of other realities that are happening simultaneously in your life. You always have something to be grateful for, and shifting your focus to whatever that is will have an immediate positive impact on your overall chemistry. It isn't mystical, it's not spiritual, you don't need candles, and you don't need a medium to help you talk to the dead.

The following is a simple exercise that I do when I first wake up in the morning, right before I open my eyes. I make sure that my attention is not on an obsession or on something negative. I think about how amazing it is to be alive. I go through my own list of things that I'm grateful for. It's not always easy to do this: Sometimes I have to wrestle with the thoughts that pop it into my head.

Doing this will be a different experience for everyone. Some people have very frightening and debilitating problems, and some people are in extraordinary pain. But no matter where you are in life, it's advisable to reach deep and find something to be grateful for. Think about that thing and embrace it.

That thought process is a thing that will save you. It's a thing that can lift you out of the muck and mire. There are many exercises that can instill gratitude in your life, but I recommend very highly that you work on a detailed gratitude list when you have a clear state of mind.

Reach deep into your history when you do. In my gratitude list, I wrote down some of the following things: I'm grateful that I was stubborn at different stages of my life, because I was able to resist lines of thought that were not enlightened. I'm grateful for my mind. I'm grateful for the ocean. I'm grateful for having survived many dangerous things. I'm grateful that I have the ability to let go of silly nonsense that doesn't serve me well. I'm grateful for the people I have in my life.

Working on gratitude is not a New Age way of facing a difficult life. Gratitude is something that has been practiced in beautiful ancient cultures since the beginning of time.

They spent a lot of their time being thankful for great lessons from their ancestors. For the abundance that the earth provided, for beautiful campfires, for birds that sang beautiful songs, for the lakes and the rivers and the oceans that provided them with the most important substances for their survival. They spent much of their time in a state of gratitude, and they had respect for the good things that the world provided them with.

Hopefully you see where I'm going with this. Gratitude is not something that was invented by the 12-step recovery founders. It's not a faddish technique that a pop psychology guru dreamed up. Rather it's one of the cornerstones of the mindsets of great people from great societies. It's something we should treasure.

I'm grateful for a beautiful oak tree that gives me shade. If I were a flesh eater I would be grateful to the animal that gave its life for my meals. If we lack gratitude, it just means that we're being grumpy. We're being agitated teenagers that refuse to see the truth. And that makes us really unhappy; in the absence of deliberate gratitude, we experience deliberate frustration, anger and negativity.

Sometimes we feel those emotions because something bad is happening. And when we're young, we don't have the mental fortitude to shift our focus—our mental strength isn't developed yet. That's typical among young people. But many adults lack the necessary skills and strengths to shift focus as well.

It doesn't seem popular or fashionable in our society to try to see the good in things that on the surface seem negative. For example, on a rainy day my mother will say, "It's a disgusting day—it's horrible." She fills her mind with negativity because the rain is inconvenient for her, or sometimes a rainy day just makes her feel sad. She hasn't habituated herself to just say, "Wow, it's raining! All the plants will get water, and everything that eats plants will be fed."

You can view putting this mindset into place as an exercise, or as a game that you engage in. You learn to place your attention and your focus on something that will make you see the world in a way that makes you happy. I can't force you into that state of mind—you have to be willing to be in it and be proactively taking steps to get yourself there.

If you're reading these words and you agree with them, then stop and be grateful for the words. Be grateful for the trees that gave paper for this book. Be grateful for something. Gratitude is absolutely essential. It will play a vital role in your attempts to do well with weight control, attain good mental and physical health, improve your relationships with others, and adopt an incredibly exciting, rewarding, and satisfying lifestyle.

111. How to Meditate

Learning how to meditate is the most advanced step in any psychological healing process. I'd like to discuss the concept and give some guidance regarding the practice. I will be making another book available that will provide greater detail about it, but you will find the information that I give you in this section to be very helpful in the short term.

To me, meditation is not a spiritual activity—rather it is 100% mental.

Meditation is not magic. We are not looking for contact with ancient gods, nor are we freeing a genie from a lamp. In the process of meditation, you don't need a special handshake, code words, or ancient chants to gain control over the mind.

You do need a lot of practice, though. Maybe even an entire lifetime of it. This is the case because as you explore the mind, your true deep consciousness begins to surface. Meditation then becomes a progression with no end, and with no limit to where you can journey with a still mind, free from obsessions and uncontrollable thinking.

No matter what stage in life you are in, it is not too early or too late to practice meditation. You can sit still or move about—it doesn't matter. As long as you can concentrate on a single thing (not two or more things), you're meditating.

Meditation is prolonged, single-minded concentration. It simply means that you make a conscious decision during a point in time to be totally present with the moment. Focus on one thing, such as the flow of your breathing—all other thoughts should cease.

At first it's normal to not believe that meditation will do a single thing to make life better. But among many other benefits, meditation will help you to stop drifting backward to previous moments or falling forward into anticipated future moments.

There's one other place we can drift—that is to nowhere. We drift to the nothingness of each and every thought as it arrives. It's in contrast to our tendency to think obsessively all day from morning to night.

We are engaged in our life's drama. We can't separate our lives from our thoughts. The ultimate truth in reality is in contrast to the fiction we create.

Meditation saved my ass, and it can save yours. But it will be a very different path for you than it has been for me. My mom didn't carry you in her belly, so you can't be exactly who I am. We are different, but we are similar.

It will take years for you to achieve the full benefits of meditation. You start slow, as if you were in an amusement park driving a bumper car. Then, over your time, you will develop into a Lockheed Martin F-35 fighter jet! In doing so, you will move at your own pace. You can start off with meditating while walking, while swimming, while running, while lifting weights, or while doing just about any other activity.

I explained to my sister, who is 53 years old and 34 years sober, that meditation doesn't begin with a marathon event. The ability to sit quietly and not get bored or frustrated takes time, and that's the purpose. The mastery of the mind is to be able to walk yourself past boredom and frustration and be in the present moment with yourself. This may take a lot of time.

If you watch children when they're doing homework or something else that's boring to them, it's amazing to see their level of frustration during their boredom. It's like watching someone go through physical pain. They may cry from boredom, or they may act up and do destructive things.

And us grownups are far worse—because the things that we can do that are destructive are far more dangerous than what a child can do. We can self-destruct, or we can destroy the world around us.

Meditation can begin just by simply being able to stay present with your breath and your footsteps when you're walking. Or you can meditate while participating in the practice of yoga. Staying totally concentrated and focused on the posture is good training.

First of all, you have a distraction, which is the physical posture. Some of the postures are difficult to do if your mind is drifting. Yet even with the difficult postures, people still find ways to drift away from where they are, because that's how they've conditioned themselves to be. It's a lack of proper conditioning of the mind.

People find it hard to do something that requires patience and concentration, especially if they don't see the endgame. Some ask, do you really believe that people throughout all of history who seemed to be tranquil and nonviolent would waste a lot of time practicing something of no value?

I think it's the misconception that meditation is only for the highly developed person, the monk, the yoga master, or the New Age hippie. It's just a western way of looking at something totally backwards. We ignore something that indigenous ancient cultures have been using since the beginning of mankind as a way of having clarity and understanding.

In the advanced practice of meditation (hold onto your socks, because this is true), you'll just meditate to join the collective consciousness of humanity. We meditate to be able to contemplate all of creation and how what is going on in our lives is relevant.

• •

Focused meditation is, metaphorically speaking, the ultimate mirror to see what is going on inside your mind. As we become more skilled, we become more able to change things in our inner worlds.

• •

One of the first things we change is our inability to tolerate frustration. We change the constant need to think about things and do things as a condition to feeling complete. We can find pleasure and joy in stillness. If one desires, they can make the focus of a meditation to just being present and feeling a sense of being.

Meditation sessions can be extremely powerful experiences. And they represent more of the truth than does the ordinary and sometimes ridiculous way that we live as modern people. In the modern world, we focus on temporal things such as accumulation of too many possessions—such things are of little value in the long run.

And we unproductively obsess on other things of little or no value—the passage of time, the impressions that people have of us, etc. We don't really have an understanding of the nature of our existence—and this is metaphysical immaturity.

Meditation is a way to unravel all of what I described. In its simplest form, it can just be a way to be present with something that you're doing in that moment, such as breathing.

Another way I describe meditation is as follows: Imagine yourself driving and you're completely distracted by your cell phone, putting on makeup, or tuning the radio. You're far more likely to get into an accident because you're distracted. Imagine a racecar driver being distracted by a cell phone. Without the 110% focus required, the result would be a crash into a wall at 200 miles per hour.

We do the things that we're doing better if we are focused on what we're doing. And what we are doing while we are here is life. It's an unsatisfactory situation if we become distracted by nonsense while we're in the process of life.

The first step in meditation is to come to believe that it is something of value. The second step is to not avoid it either because it sounds boring or because we think we don't have the time. That's not true. Anyone can find three minutes a day to concentrate on breathing. You can be walking, cycling, doing yoga, swimming, or lifting weights. Just practice being in the moment while doing so.

Make yourself into an observer of your own thought processes. You are a lifeguard in a sense; you have to bring your thought processes back to the present moment when they begin to drift.

In this age of information, there are countless numbers of videos on YouTube that can teach meditation in a variety of effective ways. There are an endless number of books. Develop your interest in the subject with fervor, because it will surely save you. Meditation is an incredibly effective tool for dispersing anxiety and stress.

And meditation will get easier as you practice three minute exercises. Over time, your exercises will become 10 minute ones with no problem at all. Within a fairly short time, you will not dread sitting in meditation—you will crave it. I promise.

Lastly, in the context of working with some type of addictive behavior such as overeating, undereating, or being addicted to junk food, the 12 steps of Alcoholics Anonymous can be very helpful. You just need to replace the word "alcohol" with "food." (Also, be aware that if your specific issue is overeating, that a 12-step program called "Overeaters Anonymous" is available worldwide and online.) The 11th step in 12-step programs suggests that a person seek out prayer and meditation to improve their own conscious contact with their higher power.

There's a lot to unpack in that step to be able to understand it adequately. And it's interesting that 12-step programs that were created only a relatively short time ago historically understood the value of meditation as being crucial in self-help disciplines.

Remember that meditation does not have to be a religious practice, unless you want it to be and/or need it to be. Meditation is an intellectual unfolding. It is a concentrated effort to streamline your thought processes and awaken your consciousness. Concepts that we talk about in this regard can take years to come into focus. But do the work, and you will reap the benefits. Perhaps slowly, but surely. Once again, I promise you this.

112. Meditation Is a Long-Term Practice

If at first you cannot meditate, try, try, try again until you succeed. If you are ready to start, it's amazingly easy. The only character attribute that you need is patience. If you feel discomfort in a seated position because it's too painful, then start on your back.

The first meditation will be the practice of just making it to your yoga mat or cloth. Lay on your back and tell yourself, "I am here to meditate." Then go to sleep if you want to, or close your eyes and drift off into all of the world's problems. Then, make a promise to yourself that you're going to show up at the same place, at the same time 24 hours later, roll out some kind of mat, and try again for just two or three minutes that day. Remember to say, "I am here to meditate."

You can try to meditate on these days and times that you come to the mat, or you can just doze off and figure out all of the world's crises as you sleep. Whenever your meditation practice becomes difficult, fall back on this 2-3 minutes per day exercise.

Eventually what we're looking to find is the ability to lay on our backs for two to five minutes and follow our own breathing. Every time a thought comes into our head about anything other than the breath, we simply don't invite it in. We do whatever we can, using whatever technique we can, to muster strength to push distracting thoughts far away. But we must be engaged in the struggle to create silence in our minds.

Please Note: Discussion on meditation can take many twists and turns into metaphysical topics and complex philosophical ponderings regarding the nature of true self and consciousness. I enjoy talking about meditation but find writing about it to be very difficult. This is the case for two reasons. One reason is because describing certain things to individuals who haven't experienced them is a formidable challenge in itself. Another reason is that certain things of many different kinds simply defy explanation. A few examples of things other than meditation that are difficult to describe include the taste of chocolate, complex mathematics, and the physics behind gravity.

All of the safety and positive emotional power that humans are seeking can be found in the stillness of meditation. And like most good things, reaping its benefits usually requires some focused effort along with a good deal of practice time. You can learn more about meditation, similar practices, and other positive lifestyle changes in the supporting articles available on the *www.goodsugar.life* website.

113. Apology Accepted

Problems in our relationships with people are among the many things that cause anxiety, pressure, distraction, and blockage with our emotions. In turn, those things may lead us to want to reach out for something unhealthy to soothe us.

I feel as if I've been reaching out for things to soothe me my entire life instead of reaching inward. But in the course of my work, my writing, and my self-discovery, I've seen that I need to look at my relationships with people every day and figure out where I have made mistakes.

When I apologize to people, I feel like my relationships stay inside their proper boundaries, not causing chaos or not blowing up in my face. So I have to say that it's for selfish reasons that I very often have to go to people and say, "I'm sorry for that thing that I did, please forgive me."

When you're married and have children, you likely have to apologize every single day of your life. You have to keep track of a lot of apologies. This is yet another of many reasons that you really need to keep a journal. A key journal entry consists of making a list of people that you need to make amends with.

This is emphasized in the writings of 12-step recovery as well as in a number of ancient philosophies. Step 8 in 12-step recovery states, "Made a list of all persons we had harmed, and became willing to make amends to them all." And step 9 reads, "Made direct amends to such people wherever possible, except when to do so would injure them or others."

I also believe that it's important to make a list of the people who have harmed us. It's important to understand that in addition to harm that we have caused, things were also dumped on us, especially in our formative years. One of many reasons we feel anxiety and stress is because we feel that we've been wronged in different ways.

It would be nice if everyone in the world adhered to practices similar to steps 8 and 9 of 12-step programs, coming to us saying "I'm sorry for that thing I did, I was wrong." That's not going to happen anytime soon, though. But it's still incumbent upon us to behave in a way that prevents us from creating more chaos. If you've done something to harm somebody, you must learn to utter the words "I'm sorry" in order to make things right.

This will have a positive, lasting effect on our ability to stay clean from addictive behavior of any kind. So saying "I'm sorry" in the context of arresting addictive behavior is admittedly a little self-centered. We are motivated to apologize to others for the purpose of improving ourselves. Later on in life that might change: You may become completely selfless in your apologies, making those apologies just because it's the right thing to do.

But in any case, you must be very aware that making an apology that will hurt the other person is completely unacceptable. This is so whoever the other person might be—a spouse, parent, child, coworker, boss, friend, or stranger. You must determine whether or not the apology would cause more harm than good.

You should first make a private list of those who you owe apologies to. You should then share that list with someone you trust. Following that, you can determine the next course of action. You can consider each item on your list and decide if an apology would be helpful or harmful.

The next right thing to do is to make amends to those you have wronged. Doing so will often free you from guilt. Guilt is a very strong motivator that can cause you to act out in negative behaviors such as overeating and using destructive, addictive substances.

It's also important to make the list of people that you think have harmed you. You should describe how they harmed you and why you think they did so. Some of the harm that was done to us might be such that we should confront our perpetrator. We might need to pray and meditate beforehand in such situations.

Forgiveness begins with a decision to forgive, but it may take years to create it. We may need time to come to an understanding of how someone could have wronged us. It may take considerable time to process our feelings to come to a place of forgiveness. But doing so is essential: Asking for forgiveness is a really important aspect of humanity's collective healing.

Becoming the type of person that can say you're sorry promptly after making mistakes moves you closer toward building your character into a fortress. It's a way to preserve valuable relationships and it's a way of reducing the number of chaotic events that occur in your life. Repentance and forgiveness are very important in developing the ability to hold mental stillness and the feeling of freedom from suffering.

114. Helping Others and Being of Service

Service to others is not an afterthought. It's not optional. It's deeply embedded into our minds and bodies—it's part of how we were designed as a species.

Help others who suffer. The first time I ever read the step referring to this in the 12 steps of Alcoholics Anonymous I wanted nothing to do with it. I was 15 years old. The step reads, "Having had a spiritual awakening as the result of these steps, we tried to carry this message to alcoholics, and to practice these principles in all our affairs."

As a teenage boy I thought this step stunk of religiosity and weird spiritualism. I reluctantly worked this step in various stages of my life because I knew that the step would help keep me sober. But looking back, I see that my attitude showed how arrogant and self-centered I was. Later in life I realized that the step is a very sophisticated psychological endeavor for a number of reasons.

One of the reasons is the benefit derived from knowledge transfer. I learned that by attempting to teach something to someone else I had a better chance of absorbing it myself at a deep level. So in helping another learn, I teach myself as well. In teaching another person how not to suffer, you teach yourself how not to suffer.

We must realize that we are all extremely self-centered people. We are constantly obsessed with ourselves and our own problems. Sometimes the only way to get our obsessions out of our own heads is to do something for others. In doing so, we take our eyes off of ourselves for a certain period of time, and it's a good thing to do so. So it's a distraction, but a very healthy one.

• •

Being of service to others really serves you at the same time. This is because ultimately you are connected to everyone and everything. You create a very positive wavelength in your mind when you are looking out for your brothers and sisters.

• •

So it's a bit of a paradox: Acts of service to others are both selfish and selfless. They are selfish in a good way (if that's possible) because you are aware of the fact that helping others will benefit you. But the real benefit occurs when you do acts of service to others in a spirit of selflessness—when you invest your own time, energy, and at times finances when it's somewhat inconvenient and uncomfortable to do so.

So, it's possible and even good to do good things just because it makes you happy and helps you in your recovery. But it's better to do good things just for the sake of doing those good things. The more you impact people's lives in a positive way, especially in the realm of overcoming addictions, the better you feel about yourself. The better we feel about ourselves as a foundation, the more we are willing to do the hard psychological work inherent in pursuing our own happiness.

There are literally millions of forms these acts of service can take. You could reach out to someone with a problem similar to yours, talking to them while giving support, positive messages, and steps to follow. You could take trips overseas to help those in extreme poverty. You could do local community service of some type, or start a nonprofit organization based on ideas you might have. The list really is endless.

I personally don't believe that this type of service is encompassed in preaching of the gospel of any particular religion, although some will benefit from receiving such information. Being of service is allowing a person to be where they're at and offering them help in a way that they can digest it and in a way that they can apply it.

To summarize, benefits that come from actions taken while helping others are many. **Nurturing of a strong sense of purpose, providing inspiration to others, making new friends, and improving a wounded self-image are but a few of those benefits.** Engage wholeheartedly in helping others while you are participating in recovery, and meditate and reflect on the many benefits that will come to you as you do so.

Nothing takes you out of your own problems and negative feelings better than getting up and doing something truly helpful for others. There are no negative side effects to this activity. There is always some person or some creature needing your help, attention, care, teaching, concern, and service.

Help people in ways that they need. I don't consider crusaders proselytizing people, attempting to get them to embrace new religions, to be performing acts of service. People need to have their emotional and physical needs met. But calling a friend who has problems, listening to the problems and comforting them, certainly constitutes an act of service. Taking an elderly family member for a walk on the boardwalk and talking with them about life is service. Being kind and being present with your children is service.

There are countless opportunities throughout the day to interact with people in a service-oriented way. And as was mentioned earlier, service makes you feel great emotionally and even physically, providing you with measurable health benefits in the process. In addition to that, service will raise your physical and emotional "vibrations" and eventually move you into a higher state of consciousness.

PART 7
INTEGRATING AND INCORPORATING THIS PROGRAM INTO YOUR LIFE

115. Make a Daily Ritual of Returning to Your Shrine to Recommit to Your Recovery

A critical aspect of mastering one's addictions, especially food-related ones, is to set aside a minimal amount of time every single day, seven days a week, that you dedicate to something that you call a self-help practice.

That dedicated time can be while you're exercising, during a yoga class, while going to a 12-step meeting, while on a daily walk, during your personal writing time, while going to temple or church for worship, while meditating, while cooking, while cleaning, while chopping wood, or while doing one of many other things.

This is your daily reprieve and your commitment to your abstinence, health and wellness desires, time improvement, and other things that you are actively doing to better yourself.

When you make this time a conscious time to think about your overall recovery needs, goals, and methods, you are reminding yourself every day of what you are committed to doing. It will keep you from forgetting or pulling away from your ultimate purpose of recovery and self-help—to stay clean, to abstain from acting out behavior, and to abstain from practices that are harmful to your health and well-being.

During the 2020 pandemic, my times for dedication to my healthy lifestyle practices were my yoga practices and my preparations prior to them. Before my practice, I put away my office-related things. I straightened up the home office. I took a quick shower to reset and refresh my mind. I set up the yoga mat and lay on my back for 3-5 minutes to relax. I checked in with myself to see what extra stuff might be buzzing around in my head—I tried to reset if there was something distracting in there. I thought about my gratitude items, I thought about how important it was that I was sober. I thought about how strong I would be in that day's yoga session.

This was and still is my ritual and routine. I feel out-of-whack completely if I miss a day. On my days off from this, I have to sit and meditate for a minimum of 10 minutes, which always leads to 10 more minutes. Once I sit to meditate, I do not get up for at least 30 minutes.

When I was younger and new in recovery, my similar tribute to recovery time was bike riding, going to the gym, and sports of some kind. I communicated to myself quite well through motion and athletics. I would work out obsessions this way, I would pray, and I would relieve stress and commit myself to the lifelong practice of being sober.

This is a surefire way to set up lasting recovery. Not only do you clear your mind and dedicate the exercise practice to your health, wellness, and addiction recovery, but you also get a good workout in. Two-for-one!

Make it to the mat every day. Make it to your shrine. Make it to your altar and stay interested and committed to the noble cause. Seven days per week, no breaks.

116. This Program Is a New Power

Granted, weight loss and radical dietary changes are very difficult lifestyle adaptations. This book is not about products for sale or exaggerated claims about dietary fixes. Rather, it is a collection of researched facts, informed opinions, and pieces of advice regarding positive dietary changes.

Through years of observation, I have formed many personal conclusions about food. My mentors taught me how to look at the chemistry of nutrition as it relates to the body. I now investigate and explore existing science in this field in order to create food-related hypotheses, which I then attempt to prove throughout the course of my life.

After observing hundreds of test subjects over the years, it has become extremely clear that when a person of any race, color, creed, denomination, age group, or lifestyle eliminates processed food from their diet, they see immediate improvements in their body chemistry. It is amazing to witness this among such a diverse group.

The days of large numbers of people mocking the truth that clean, healthy nutrition is vital to maintaining a strong immune system are coming to an end. We now live in a day and age where all reputable scientists agree to that.

There may be detractors, but you have to consider the sources. Some strong proponents of harmful diets who consider themselves to be experts push diets that they want to keep for themselves. There is much misinformation and foolishness being perpetuated. I'm aware of many books on the subject of recovering from cancer that are 99% spot on until they discuss the subject of protein.

Everything I have observed and am willing to discuss is not meant to be judgmental or critical of others; it is merely an attempt to help people who are struggling with, or looking to improve, their biological chemistry.

117. Taking Ownership and Dietary Transition

The problem with commercialized diets and plans is that they are dependent on other people trying to do the work for you. By that I mean that by attempting to follow a given plan to the letter, a user is to some degree depending on the individual or organization to do the hard work that only he or she can do. The user has to go through difficult moments when abstaining from compulsive overeating or eating junk food.

But the user also has to take complete ownership of the process of weight loss, and that requires personal responsibility. Many plans and diets, especially fad diets, don't help users face up to their own unwise lifestyle choices.

••

There isn't a magic formula or secret to truly sustainable weight loss. But, as I previously discussed, there are a number of things that one can implement that over time, possibly over a relatively short time, will lead to significant weight loss.

••

One is eating a wholesome plant-based diet. Another is increasing physical activity. And not surprisingly, another is restriction of caloric intake (difficult at first, but the intake restriction becomes considerably easier once one transitions to a much healthier diet).

Transition is a key factor. If you change your lifestyle, your cravings for unhealthy food will surface. So will emotions that trigger unhealthy eating patterns. But these things can be overcome.

You may need to go through a detoxification diet. Doing so will make it so that toxins will be removed from your body, via your bloodstream and your butt. This detoxification gets rid of necrotic rotting food that lodges itself in your digestive system.

Many people overlook the fact that they must seek to improve their mental and emotional health as they are seeking to lose weight. Striving to heal wounds connected to anxiety, unhappiness, and repressed feelings is a must, because these things are major causes for poor dietary choices.

But the wounds can be healed, provided that essential steps are taken concurrently with better dietary choices. Meditation, yoga, prayer, talking with others, therapy, journaling, and research are among the steps that will help immeasurably with long-term weight loss success.

It bears repeating: Those steps are essential.

118. A Final Pitch on Veganism and Avoiding Processed Food

I am not a "vegan preacher." My platform has always been to explain to others to first and foremost eliminate processed food before changing other dietary patterns. I have explained the plant-based lifestyle in the previous chapters, and I understand that there is controversy among people about whether or not we need flesh foods.

But, as a vegan, the further away I go from eating any type of animal flesh, meat, or secretion, the more outlandish it seems to me that we, as humans, choose to eat these foods. It's also outlandish that we have conditioned ourselves to believe that they are not only appetizing, but necessary for our survival. There is absolutely nothing more bizarre than the assumption that eating meat is required for a healthy diet.

The only thing as comparatively bizarre is the consumption of semi-edible, synthetic, and processed substances created by people who have zero interest in your health, and who have learned to exploit people who have food addictions and food ignorance.

119. Food Industry Issues

The problem in the professional food industry is that people are constantly trying to tailor diets to individuals with extremely poor eating habits. They then try to apply those same dietary concepts to people with healthy biological chemistry, and those people then become unhealthy.

I want you to picture your diet as a bridge connecting two pieces of land divided by water. With the right engineering and building materials, the structure can be built stronger and lighter. With poor engineering and heavy building materials, the bridge must be built with extra considerations just to support its own weight, not to mention the weight of the vehicles crossing the bridge.

This metaphor is especially relevant to your diet if you are consuming foods of two particular categories: 1) Those that are extremely resistant to digestion, 2) Those that require so much work to be converted into energy that you need to eat more of them simply for digestion, instead of for their nutrients. Again, one tremendous bodily function is that of healing and detoxification, but the person's diet must support this.

When people look at their caloric intake, they generally do not take into consideration that the body requires calories just to digest food. They must keep in mind the direct impact that different foods have on the overall immunological system.

Certain foods that people consume, processed foods created by the food industry in particular, are simply garbage. Our bodies were never meant to eat heavily processed or synthetic foods. Human bodily chemistry has never adapted to support the waste they create or to compensate for the lack of nutrients from these products.

120. Energy of Food

Connect to the energy of food. Not just the literal energy but the low frequency energies, such as electrical forces and the most subtle force of food; the foods' residual spiritual energies that are connected to the divine intelligence of all creation.

You are the very food that you eat—it is a part of you. You are connected to everything, whether you feel this or not. Even if you can't make out the subtle vibrations of these energies and subtle forces, they affect us all to some degree.

121. Abstinence

Abstain from anything that is bad for you. Any food with a high degree of negative effect on the chemistry, any food that does not have an 80% degree of being supremely beneficial to us, is not a food we should be eating.

Alcohol, lifestyle mistakes such as smoking, high levels of stress, and ordinary dietary mistakes such as simply exceeding the amount of calories required for daily function—all of these should be abstained from. For the ultimate diet, abstinence, not moderation, from things that are bad for you is what should be practiced.

Abstinence from overeating and eating junk food is an important accomplishment, and as such it should be measured and recorded. When a person starts on their food recovery journey, that is day one. It is an important part of the psychological component that we count days, and then months, and then years that we are free of our negative behaviors.

These milestones in recovery are our anniversaries—celebrate them (but without chocolate cake or ice cream). By keeping track of time, we make the continuous achievement of remaining abstinent more important to us. When we keep track, beginning with writing down our start dates, we are less likely to have relapses and less likely to minimize them if they happen.

And we can take great pride in these anniversaries that we experience. Not with a selfish, unhealthy pride, but with a sense of gratitude and happiness upon reflecting on the very positive and life-giving steps that we've taken on our journeys.

122. Elimination and Irregularity

All books on nutrition in general and weight loss in particular should give some information about the elimination of your body's waste. It's an important factor in nutrition and weight loss, and I'm not sure why it's often neglected.

It's not difficult to comprehend why going to the bathroom on a regular basis has an enormous impact on how we lose weight, as well as on other vital things such as how we sleep, the state of our moods, and our overall chemistry.

There are three locations in the home which are of the highest value: (1) the kitchen; (2) the bedroom; and (3) the bathroom. Each room is an important part of your overall health. We all sleep, eat, eliminate and bathe.

I figured out a long time ago that I undervalued the time I spent in the bathroom. I distracted myself because using the bathroom is boring. I realized the importance of going to that room empty handed. No phones, no books, no distractions. Some people love a good read while they're on the can. I have learned how to sit quietly when it's potty time and focus. I focus on my diet and focus on my mood. I am grateful for my health and this is the time to think about it.

In the split second before I flush, I have to look and rate my poo. This is normal and this is critical to self-help and self-healing. We have to know for sure what's going on with the waste removal system and plumbing within us. I suggest to anyone who is working on heightening their overall consciousness, use these moments to focus and unravel distractions.

If the food you eat backs you up so that you have difficulty going to the bathroom, that alone can make you feel very anxious and unhappy. Unpleasant physical sensations such as painful mosquito bites, back pain, and a myriad of other things will definitely affect your overall outlook on life. If you've been backed up and irregular for years, it's not surprising if it has had a negative impact on your emotions and the way that you see the world.

The most common physical emotion that results from being irregular is anxiety. Anxiety is really just a vibration that begins with a thought and a concept in the head. It's telling you that something might be wrong, or maybe there's something to be afraid of. In the case of being backed up, there is something wrong and there is something to be concerned about. Therefore, your body is signaling you correctly, and your responding by expressing anxiety and/or concern is appropriate.

Some of us are physically more sensitive than others, and if that's the case our feelings are more likely to physically affect us. Other people may have very strong constitutions and not be as easily affected, even when experiencing unbelievable amounts of stress, but we should not compare ourselves with others.

I've heard a number of brilliant people speak on these matters. Some people tie a constipation problem to a person's difficulty in letting go of things; emotional things, physical things, or the excrement itself. It's difficult to find scientific proof of this.

It's certainly logical that if you carry different emotional problems, then you may be constipated to some degree as a result. But if you work on your emotional issues and clean up your diet, there's no reason that you shouldn't have a large bowel movement at least once a day. When you get really healthy, you'll be able to poop at least twice a day.

But there is a second part to the equation. You could be eating a great diet, but still have many emotional disruptions; fear, anxiety, depression, sadness, anger, resentment, etc. Such feelings would likely create constipation or irregularity. So, sometimes the first cause could be that your diet is off. It then affects your regularity, which in turn affects your emotions. And at other times the reverse is true, in which case your emotions are out of balance, which in turn affects your regularity.

There's no escaping how the body and the mind interact with each other in every way. That is why only a holistic approach works on an ultimate plan of self-healing, diet and self-improvement. In other words, you can't just work on your body and ignore your emotional world. Nor can you just work on your emotional world and ignore your body. Both must be attended to simultaneously.

This section is not intended to diagnose bowel disorders—there are far too many types. And it's nothing to be ashamed of if you're having emotional issues that sometimes affect your ability to eliminate. This happens to everyone at times.

There are many reasons why someone's regularity could be off. I would advise anyone who hasn't been able to improve their regularity after a reasonable amount of time attempting to address the problem through diet, exercise, and work on their emotional issues to consult a physician or specialist.

123. Dietary Issues and Irregularity

What type of diet can make a person constipated or irregular?

First and foremost, understand that a diet that is high in protein is not optimal for taking a shit.

If you're constipated, don't panic. Don't take drugs. Don't take pills. Don't hang upside down from your feet.

Start off by making sure you have two large leafy green salads every day. You shouldn't have them at nighttime, because that can clog you. It can also cause gas or indigestion. You can eat a salad for breakfast. In time, you'll begin to crave it.

It's only because of marketing and social conditioning that salad does not sell for breakfast. Salad doesn't look like what we were programmed to believe is a morning food. But I would definitely recommend a large, leafy green salad for breakfast to get the day going.

The salad can even contain some citrus fruits. They are very compatible for digestion with leafy greens. You can enjoy a blended smoothie that combines both greens and a variety of fruits.

Take a look at what you have visualized as being good for breakfast since you were a kid. People think of eggs, waffles (which are basically sugary pastries), pancakes, bread, doughnuts, muffin, bagels, and things like bacon as morning foods.

The waffles and pastries are mostly just refined starchy carbohydrates—the worst type of carbohydrates. The best carbohydrates are those that occur naturally in wholesome foods such as fruits and vegetables. Your metabolism has an entirely different reaction to naturally occurring carbohydrates rather than processed carbohydrates.

Processed carbohydrates are extremely concentrated sugars; this means that there are a lot of sugar molecules in a very tiny space. Everything is amplified. Your body chemistry's reaction to something so concentrated is much more extreme. And this is not optimal.

Some people might consider a bagel with cream cheese and perhaps some smoked salmon to be a good breakfast choice. But such a breakfast would be lacking valuable minerals and vitamins. That type of food will put an extra burden on your digestive system, because it doesn't break down easily. Neither does the protein from eggs.

The toxicity of the components in a grill or pan fried bacon are disasters to body chemistry as well. They will definitely have a negative impact on your emotions and your clarity throughout your entire day. In addition to that, these cooked foods and processed foods are devoid of living enzymes and healthy probiotic bacteria, which are vital to the functioning of your bowels.

What you eat will control your energy levels, the clarity in which your brain functions, and your overall emotional world. As I stated earlier, your emotions are not just guided by what happens to you and what you think. You're also guided by how your body physically feels at any given moment.

If you start your day off with a terrible breakfast, you have in effect just jumped off a cliff. By the end of the day you will have hit the bottom of the cliff. The cliff bottom is generally in the form of cravings for different foods at nighttime when your body should be in a resting mode.

People that eat high-protein, highly concentrated food will definitely need more fiber to push that stuff out of the system. The fiber is like a broom, and it's also the thing that stimulates your body to push food through the digestive system. The insoluble fiber is part of what forms a solid stool. Other parts of the fiber are the food that good bacteria eat and need in order to live and carry out their digestive functions.

The most fibrous food we can eat comes from the plant kingdom—not from a bagel or a waffle. Plant food is the fiber that your body was expecting. If the fiber that you're getting is coming from grains in a wholesome bread, that's an option, but those grains are usually harder to digest than the fiber that comes from fruits and leafy vegetables.

124. Suggested Remedies for Irregularity

The most important remedy for elimination problems in any mammal is to consume the bitter greens—to eat lots of light green colored leafy vegetables.

All the fruits are good, but some fruits are better than others. If you like prunes, you should try plums. Plums have plenty of water in them, and when they're fresh they actually take on a new dynamic that they lose when they are dried. Other good fruits include dates, nectarines, apples, oranges, celery, pomegranate, lemon, and melon eaten by itself (not with other fruits).

Watermelon is a great bathroom remedy for four reasons: It's filled with water, it's filled with naturally-occurring sugars, it's filled with water-soluble fiber, and it contains the good bacteria that naturally aids in good health.

Taking a good probiotic may be one of the better solutions to elimination problems, because having a healthy balance of the right digestive flora is critical for proper gastronomic functionality. But if you choose to use a probiotic, you must ensure that it is a high quality product that is derived from a universally beneficial bacteria strain.

125. Keeping a Scale in the House

Ultimately it is you who is responsible for the decisions you will make and what will bring comfort into your life. Remember that happiness is a crucial part of your health.

Of the many people that I have helped in my life, I've never seen a scale make them happy over the long run. The first problem is if people become weight-obsessed, rather than focused on the big picture of their overall health. It's easy to get caught up in the attachment of losing weight rather than the attachment of changing one's lifestyle.

What I've seen is that when people use a scale, they tend to reward themselves by going back to the old eating pattern after they lose some weight. And they seem to punish themselves if they've gained weight. For those reasons alone I am not a proponent of keeping a scale at home.

On the other hand, you may be a person that needs very specific milestones to keep you going; you may be a highly competitive person, even if the competition is just with yourself.

If you choose to keep and use a scale, pay close attention as the weeks and months go by to how your victories and defeats feel.

I am totally against putting myself on a roller coaster ride. I know exactly what I need to do on a daily basis to nourish myself and to make sure that I feel good.

I use the feeling in my body and the feeling in my stomach to help me determine how my day went and what I have to work on tomorrow. I know exactly when I've eaten too much. And so I use my instincts as my own measure. I realize that what I do may seem too difficult for others, but you can do it. I encourage you to try.

126. Your Relationship With Food and Lifestyle Choices Moving Forward

I find it remarkable how much effort the western world has to put into making sure that we have the right relationship with food. It is a relatively modern phenomena that has been amplified in the last hundred years.

I imagine that the industrial age of massive farming, coupled with food preservation techniques and refrigeration, coupled with these massive supermarkets that we have, have amplified the problem. **The problem is that we are expecting ourselves to remain connected to food when we are only connected to the eating process.**

The vast majority of us do not have to handle livestock. We don't have to plant seeds and worry about rain or drought. We are completely dependent on a system to nourish us. The problem is that this system is broken, extremely dysfunctional, and corrupt. And it's well beyond the scope of my knowledge to know how to fix it.

But the reason I am bringing this to your attention is that these facts make it clear that you are mostly on your own when it comes to fixing your relationship with food.

Just look at our relationship with food and how we obtain it. Then connect the dots once again to the feelings of anxiety that most of us feel resulting from childhood experiences coupled with present situations. It's all but impossible to not fall into the trap of an eating problem.

The solution may not be as easy as starting a vegetable garden, living in the woods and following all the perfect rhythms of nature in relation to your body. Such a scenario may not be obtainable for you. But you can certainly follow one of the natural laws of a hygienic diet, which is to only eat wholesome pure foods free of toxins.

At the risk of sounding like a broken record, the most powerful and obvious thing that we can do is to abstain completely from processed foods. This alone will bring about most of the solutions to all of our dietary problems. I truly believe that if all human beings adopted this lifestyle, it would also heal some of the destructive patterns that cause harm to our great earth.

The planet has become a dumpsite because of a way of thinking that mirrors our way of thinking regarding our diet. If you adapt a more wholesome diet over the next few years, you will likely have a desire to cleanse your share of the planet. You will have a desire to live on a healthy planet as well as in a healthy body. Your body will become a place that you enjoy being in—a comfortable and familiar place to live.

In the course of this book, I've explained many things that one should do in order to overcome poor eating choices. It's my hope that you are encouraged and committed to continuing to pursue a healthy lifestyle free of bondage to food addiction or bad eating patterns.

But that might not be the case. You may be discouraged that so much work, particularly at the psychological level, is necessary. But it is, and all your hard work will pay off many times over.

I need to describe some things about the consequences of not taking the necessary steps to win your battle. The best way that I can do so is to describe my own bad experiences that occurred when I neglected to take the necessary actions of the recovery process.

127. Get Into Therapy

I mentioned therapy at some length earlier. I am deliberately separating thoughts on it in different sections in the book because repetition is critical for this subject.

I need to reiterate some of the basic concepts of therapy. You may already be a proponent of therapy and be participating in it. If so, my suggestion is to discuss with your therapist the importance of shifting the focus of your sessions to your relationship with food for a time. That doesn't mean that you should use a therapist as your nutritionist. What I do mean by this is that we have a web of emotions that are linked in to our food behaviors. Looking closely at our relationship with food throughout our life can unlock some potentially hidden mysteries about what happened to us as children.

Successful therapy is dependent on the style of the therapist and your participation in it. To benefit from therapy you have to feel safe to express a range of difficult emotions such as anger, rage, sadness, sorrow, fear, and others. A therapist has to be so many different things to a client if therapy is to be effective. It's important that a therapist has vast knowledge on the subjects of clients' needs. Good therapists must also have a great deal of experience in overcoming the adversities of their own lives.

I like therapists who aren't afraid to say judgemental shit. I like a therapist to pause me and say, "Hey Marcus, what you just said was nonsense." I don't need someone to to just sit there listening to me regurgitate and spew the events of my life. If I'm being an asshole, I need a service that will help me stop being an asshole. I need to be called up and called out; that's what I respond to.

In the old days we might've had witch doctors or shamans, or just family and close friendship relationships. But our modern day problems have become exponentially more complex. And I think it's a signal of good progress that now there's a field of science regarding sitting with a virtual stranger and talking about problems. But we can waste a lot of time in therapy skirting around the real problems.

I've found that my problems are related to my coming from an abusive, shitty childhood home that was broken and filled with lots of absurd behavior. Sometimes just using a therapist to mention these things has had a very therapeutic effect of dissolving my denial systems. My best therapists have always been mentors, not just good listeners.

I've learned that in order for me to survive my childhood, I had to build up all kinds of defenses for myself. But now, as an adult, these defenses have not served me. They did the exact opposite—they blocked me. I'm not going to spend the rest of my life in denial about my childhood, and I'm not going to resist the available therapies that are available to help me move through these things much quicker. Good therapy will promote rapid change. Good therapy can help you resist addictive, toxic behavior.

Some people are hesitant to get involved in therapy because they think it's expensive. Excuses such as that come from fear and a lack of knowledge. You can find affordable therapy if you research options. Even if you're flat broke, you can find a therapist to take on your case pro bono or offer you services on a sliding scale.

Group therapy is highly effective as long as it's facilitated by someone who knows what they're doing. Group therapy is also less expensive than individual therapy. In my opinion, it's as effective or even more so than one-on-one therapy. (That's the subject of an entire book, which I intend to write at some point.)

The most progress that I've made in my life has been during times that I've consistently participated in therapy. My wife and I have a great marriage and continue therapy to keep things in harmony. We're at the stage in therapy now where the prime focus is in marital problems. Our therapist is a wonderful teacher, and she gives us great information about human nature and how our brain functions. Our therapy sessions are like crash courses in basic and advanced psychology.

It's wonderful to me, because I pick up on information and store it. And then if there's disarray with my wife, I have information to fall back on. If some conflict builds up, I bring it up in therapy, where it's safe and where it will be resolved. With some of the more difficult issues, my therapist is my interpreter for communicating with my wife.

I've been in and out of therapy since the age of 13. My first therapist gave me a great sense of humor about my problems. We made model airplanes. We assembled model plastic replicas of guns. He was the first person who told me that my relationship with my mother wasn't very good.

I have a great image of Dr. Liebowitz etched into my mind. He was a very kind human being. He listened to my problems once a week and he showed tremendous interest. He listened to my immature teenager jokes and he giggled. He always shared a smile with me. He was the person that made a huge difference to me in that stage of my life.

Consider this analogy about therapy. If you have problems with your car and you refuse to fix them, they're likely going to cause additional problems until the car just breaks down. You need to consider your brain to be a race car that needs frequent pit stops. And today there are so many great options; one-on-one, group sessions, phone conferencing, video conferencing, and the list goes on. Participate in therapy. It will greatly accelerate your healing process.

128. Bond With Nature

In consideration of physical and psychological principles that need to be put into place to facilitate weight loss and weight control, it's appropriate to touch on the subject of connection with nature. Bonding with nature is extremely important. Doing so is how we are designed—it gets us to the very essence of our being. But don't hear what I'm not saying: I'm not suggesting that you take off your clothes and run naked through Central Park barking at the moon.

The majority of people that I've encountered in my life have a connection to nature that makes them feel grounded and happy. It has served as an important reminder to me that we all need to get close to mother nature to aid in our healing and happiness.

The longer you can surround yourself by unadulterated, wild, and powerful natural surroundings, the faster and easier our inner work on healing and wholeness will be. The sights, sounds, smells, and feelings that nature gives us have an immediate positive effect on our chemistry. It can shift the way we think if we remain present when we are experiencing nature.

That soothing, bubbly sound of the ocean wave as it's being pulled back out past the shore is a familiar sound to all of us, coming from deep, deep inside our central nervous system. We need to hear it. If we can't hear it, we need to see it. If we can't do either within our mind's eye, then we need to get face-to-face with the ocean to breathe the salty air and feel the breeze on our face. There's a miraculous internal healing power that beautiful nature inspires.

You may be a city dweller with very limited access to nature. If so, get a small plant, place it by the window, and water and nurture it. Although it will have less of an impact on you than being in the forest would, it will be considerably better than nothing at all. Caring for a plant is an important meditation.

The best natural environments are ones that have wild birds and animals that you can observe in them. Their behavior is informative to us, even if we don't understand it exactly at first. Keep watching, and cherish the moments when you do so.

Make as much time as possible to look at the night sky and count the stars. Be sure to have as many meaningful interactions as you can with trees—young ones, old ones, large ones and small ones. The desert, the forest, the ocean, the jungle, the plains, and the mountains all have personalities and qualities that show us who we are.

Human beings have domesticated themselves and have forgotten what it's like to not be confined by architecture, influenced by artificial lighting, and breathing stale recycled air. Things such as architecture may mark the pinnacle of human progress, but you and I still need to touch our feet on damp soil, warm sand, and fresh earth.

This section may sound somewhat "hippy," but it's true. And it's based on modern science as well. The University of Minnesota's website states, "Being in nature, or even viewing scenes of nature, reduces anger, fear, and stress and increases pleasant feelings. Exposure to nature not only makes you feel better emotionally, it contributes to your physical well-being, reducing blood pressure, heart rate, muscle tension, and the production of stress hormones."

Jim Robbins wrote the following for the Yale School of the Environment: "In a study of 20,000 people, a team led by Mathew White of the European Centre for Environment & Human Health at the University of Exeter, found that people who spent two hours a week in green spaces—local parks or other natural environments, either all at once or spaced over several visits—were substantially more likely to report good health and psychological well-being than those who don't. Two hours was a hard boundary: The study, published last June, showed there were no benefits for people who didn't meet that threshold. The studies point in one direction: Nature is not only nice to have, but it's a have-to-have for physical health and cognitive function."

There's no denying the value of building the necessity of spending time in nature for the purpose of therapy into your healing plan. It is as important as anything else that's covered in this book. Work at it! Work at it!

129. Sleep Is an Integral Part of Weight Loss and an Overall Sense of Well-Being

Sleep is the only rest for the giant machine that is your body; it is the time when your brain reorganizes. It's defragging the hard drive to the brain. It's also the time when you go on your own automatic dialysis: When you are in a deep sleep you are filtering your blood from garbage. Sleep is a reality change. And when you get your needed sleep, you have an opportunity to have a complete do-over from the previous day.

My wife loves to sleep and she is very ritual oriented. She goes to sleep at a set time, the shades come down, she puts essential oils in a mister, she reads from her favorite books to calm her mind, she makes the room as dark as Dracula's castle, and she has to sleep for a full eight hours.

I have irregular sleep patterns. No matter what, I wake up at the same time every day, even if I didn't go to sleep until 5 o'clock in the morning. I used to have totally insane hours back in the early days when I was building Juice Press. I was so excited and I was such a workaholic that I would get on my computer at midnight and become the company's graphic designer. I was just using those things as a way of avoiding sleep.

Sleep is really a strange activity. For creatures that are designed to be so mobile and so involved in the world, the fact that we have to turn it off every day for 8 to 10 hours seems silly. Human beings could have been designed to only need sleep every four days. We could have also been designed to only need an hour of sleep each day.

But there is a very specific program that we are biologically designed to follow. It is that for every hour we are awake, we need 30 minutes of sleep that same day—a

2 to 1 ratio. That shows you how sleep is such an integral part of our health, well-being, and our very existence.

There's a lot more going on in your sleep than just the rest of your physical body. An enormous detox process occurs when you're in a rested state. And you must provide the environment for coming to that state yourself. It's a very important part of the overall weight loss process. Your body cannot function optimally without sufficient rest.

How well you're able to get yourself to bed really is a function of your overall mental wellness, your habits, and your routines. All of your habits and routines will enable you to be able to unwind and prepare yourself for bed. As an example, if you turn on the news at 11 PM and hear about all of the world's suffering and drama, don't expect to have a good night's sleep. (It helped me to change my sleep pattern by listening to yesterday's news on the following morning.)

I stop eating a couple of hours before resting. I do this because the food itself, besides providing me with energy, has information that seeps into my consciousness and may keep me awake. If I'm extremely hungry and I find it impossible to go to bed in that state, I drink water. I squeeze a lemon in it because I find that to be very soothing, or I drink a non-caffeinated herbal tea.

Sometimes the ritual of just making tea signals to the rest of my consciousness that I'm not really hungry. I just needed some kind of routine. In order to lose weight and be healthy, you should ensure that your bed is clean and your pillows are fresh and crisp. You should also have a sleep routine. I could not overcome my sleep deprivation behavior until I created a detailed routine.

My routine is as follows: By 10 o'clock anything that I was doing that involves business is over. By 10 o'clock I have my phone plugged into a charger in a different room than where I sleep. By 10 o'clock if I'm still watching TV,

I'm only watching light hearted nonsense. I don't watch violence, I don't watch the news, and I don't watch things that require tremendous concentration and learning. In other words, I watch stupid TV.

Most nights I'm not watching TV at all. Of late, my habit is to watch educational videos on subjects that I find intriguing. Usually this gets me in the mood of being tired from boredom, or it just simply relaxes me. By 10 o'clock I am showered, and I sit somewhere quiet and review my day either by writing briefly in my Google docs or my iPhone notepad. Sometimes I just journal some of the important events of that day in my calendar.

The main thing that I try to do is be home before 10 o'clock, because if I'm out I'm stimulated. That makes me kind of bored. But I'm not really bored, because the next day I plan to be a superhero all over again. The following day I'm going to do a lot of exercise, I'm going to get a lot of creative stuff done, I'm going to work my ass off, I'm going to spend time with my family and my wife, and I'm going to do other stuff.

In order for me to function optimally, I have to admit to myself that I need sleep. I used to joke and say that sleep is the enemy of the entrepreneur. But I really meant it. As strong and as healthy and vital as I was, I realize today that it was because of my terrible sleep patterns that I might've been unnecessarily rough. If I had better sleep patterns I know I would've been more relaxed, I would've been more compassionate, and I would've been a better CEO.

I'm not reviewing this because I have regrets about it today; I just have learned my lesson. I am a sensitive, fragile, tough guy. I am made of nails, screws and hammers, but I'm also really gentle and fragile. My delicate mind needs eight hours of sleep at the right time. I can't go to sleep at 3 o'clock in the morning and wake up at 11 AM. I don't have that kind of lifestyle. I absolutely love waking up early and feeling rested.

I'm trying to train myself over time to be able to wake up at 6 AM and still get eight hours. Those are farmers hours, but they're amazing for me at this stage of my life. When I wake up early and I start my day early, it's so quiet. When I'm efficient with time I could have my critical items done before 3 PM. The point is that I'm trying to set up routines that keep me methodical and on track. This works for me because when I'm just loafing around I tend to get myself into trouble.

A good writing assignment is to create a schedule of rest that complements your schedule of work, that complements your schedule of exercise, and that complements your schedule of time with family and friends. It's probably best to set up the schedule based on the week rather than day-to-day. We obviously need eight hours of sleep every day, but you might not need to do three hours of exercise every day or spend four hours per day on the phone with your best friend to balance the calendar.

In conclusion, it is during the time that we're sleeping that our body chemistry has free reign over everything to clean up our mistakes, and to clean up the buildup of the day-to-day activity. In other words, to clean up the waste. As a matter of fact, right now it's 9:50 PM, and so this writing has to come to an end. I'm going to drink some lemon water and write in my calendar that I had a very effective day and that it's OK for me to sleep.

130. Supplements in General

First off all, I am biased because I sell supplements. Having said that, I can still teach that the best source of our nutrients is our food. Your overall health depends on how you absorb and utilize these compounds.

I do not believe in blanketing every problem with a supplement. I do not believe that a person with a clean diet and lifestyle should need to take supplements long-term. But those of us who feel we need a supplement need to know that the laboratory synthetics aren't the best option. That is because they are not the same as the supplements derived from plants; the plant-based supplements are handled and processed in a way that generally does not adulterate the final product.

The best processes for supplement production do not use potentially harmful chemical compounds to extract other compounds. In processing, low heat or no heat is better than high temperatures that can alter the structures within the compound.

Organic ingredients from a transparent supply chain is a must for all things in our diet, especially our supplements. Supplements should always bear some or all of the following symbols and text designations: "No GMOs," "Plant-based," "USDA Organic," "Non-allergenic," and "All Natural," among others.

131. Probiotic Supplements

Good bacteria, called probiotics, reside in your digestive system. They are a critical element in your overall health: They aid in weight loss, mood stability, and immunity from a host of diseases.

I have worked in the probiotics industry for a number of years, after learning about the science through my retail juice bar business.

My food mentor, Fred Bisci, introduced me to a very high-quality probiotic supplement, and a couple of years later I was packaging my own vegan probiotic supplement through an incredible company in Bulgaria. This probiotic was covered in the Wall Street Journal for being effective against common gut pathogens, and anecdotally many people have said this probiotic has vastly improved their digestion.

••

There are a number of reasons that the critical good bacteria that reside in your digestive system can go out of balance. If there is an imbalance of good bacteria, bad bacteria will proliferate and grow without being challenged.

••

A number of physical and psychological problems—including obesity, depression, lethargy, and many others—may be related to a deficiency of good bacteria in the digestive system. If you choose to take probiotics, I recommend that you choose non-dairy (plant-based) ones that use only one strain of bacteria.

132. A Glimpse Into My Personal Story

I struggled with addictions to substances, food, and toxic behavior patterns beginning in my youth and continuing throughout early adulthood. My particular addictions related to food included eating enormous amounts of all foods in general and of junk food in particular, late night eating, eating too much protein, and eating to compensate for feeling poorly. I had extreme difficulty in bottoming out in my food addictions for a number of reasons.

Approximately seven years into my sobriety, I had gotten to the point of taking no action whatsoever that would be considered part of my recovery process. My good habits had all slipped away slowly. I became lazy, complacent, apathetic, and ambivalent. In addition to that, my emotional world had become a mess.

I was depressed, anxious, lonely and bored. I was only 22 years old at the time and I had no career path and very little social life. I was clueless about life and was just getting by. I stopped my daily prayer work, likely because I did not have a substantial relationship with an object of prayer such as a God.

I let myself go. I was not practicing meditation. I had no idea how it worked. I could not sit still for 10 minutes in silence. My mind was adrift. I was not writing out my feelings. I was not in therapy. I had no support group, no AA meetings.

I had nothing but sheer grit and determination not to use drugs of any kind or drink booze. These things were not an option. This was a very dangerous place for a person with an addictive personality to wander to. However, looking back I can hardly believe that I stayed sober during the next few years.

Things changed as I entered into my ninth year of sobriety. I started a relationship with a 22-year-old model who was married to a drug dealer. She was a chain smoker and a heavy user of hard drugs (she used all drugs that were available but thankfully didn't inject them).

That nightmare relationship took me on a rollercoaster ride of madness, rejection, fear, pain, sadness, and despair. But it had to happen: I needed a tornado to rip apart my immature thought structures and get me to a new kind of emotional bottom. It worked. When that relationship was over, I was still sober and on my knees in the bathroom praying to the "universe" for help.

I jumped back into therapy in accordance with the recommendation of my sober father. Within a few short months, I started my journey and my healing process again. I learned a new set of words and recovery phrases I had never heard, resulting from my devastatingly painful and inappropriate recent relationship.

These were the words: Sex addict, romantic obsessive, anxiety disorders, and intimacy. I was able to see how my addictions were crossing over into other activities. I wasn't smoking marijuana or cigarettes but I was getting a "high" from my toxic relationship, the addiction to the drama, the obsession with the heartache, the adrenaline of the intense feelings, and the comfort of the sexual aspect when things were working out between us. I was an addict of a new kind. But I made a decision to pursue recovery in the proper way after that point.

This is what I went through. Only after much therapy, introspection, prayer, meditation, exercise, writing, and interaction with others did I get back on an effective, satisfying, and productive path of recovery.

And this is yet another reason that I wrote this book. I can't go back and change my decisions to not participate in recovery steps. But I can plead with others to not make the same mistakes. You can win your battle with weight control, but you need to fight it in the right way. Do so, and you will win!

Think of your health and wellness as if it were your car. It's your vehicle and at some point you have to get behind the wheel and drive it yourself. And a similar analogy comes from the popular apocalyptic sci-fi movie from some years back titled "The Matrix." On a couple of occasions in the film, the character Morpheus tells the lead character Neo, "I can only show you the door—you're the one who has to walk through it." I want to really encourage you to "own" the process of attaining weight control, overall health and wellness, and the by-product of satisfaction from doing so.

I wish to make one thing clear. That is this: I wrote this book as much for me as I did for you. I've used these techniques in my own life for many years and have found that they work very well.

And unfortunately I know from experience that if one "slacks off" in the path toward health, wellness, and recovery, the results will be unpleasant.

I can't envision myself straying from that particular path. But we all know that life holds many surprises and unexpected circumstances. There's always a possibility that something unexpected could come my way and cause me to stray from what I know is right. I think it's extremely unlikely that that will be the case. But should that happen, I intend to use this book and my other writings to put myself back on the right path.

To use an analogy, I consider this book and others to be maps back to my own treasure. It is a treasure to me to have obtained the clarity to examine the things that I've done to improve my own health and wellness and put them in writing.

It's a curse to fall away from the right path to health and wellness. But should that ever become the case with me, I will use my own writings, professional counseling, hard work, and a lot of help from my friends to get back on track.

As you develop and improve your own mental health, your own behavioral stability, and your own sense of awakening, I strongly encourage you to write out your own program.

Write and edit constantly; I can't stress enough how important it is to write in order to develop your own character and mental health.

I hope that you have found this book to be helpful. I intend to do future revisions of it; I consider this book and my other writings to be works in progress.

I don't consider myself to be a professional writer by any stretch of the imagination. That being the case, I find it to be very difficult to complete projects such as this one. But it's extremely rewarding to know that I have helped some people progress on the path to health and wellness. I sincerely hope that you are one of those people.

133. A Cup of Tea

In the evening when we might feel uneasy, we have to help ourselves transition from one day to the next. Pour yourself a cup of hot tea that has a happy name, a fragrant smell, and no caffeine.

Do this anytime you feel uncertain or deeply emotionally, anxious or even shut down. The tea is a symbol of soothing. The effort to make it is your hopefulness and your interest in your healing.

Sip it with intention. What does that mean? Intention is the thought behind an action. It's the purpose behind the action. We also have an intention of some kind. We can decide in many cases what the intention will be before we move forward with action.

When we do things it is smart to set our intention on doing good and not harming anything or anyone in the process. Set an intention such as, "I will let this tea make me feel happy."

134. Therapy and Determination

I started therapy when I was 13 years old. I found it very helpful even then. Today, I look back at the value that my therapy had and I realize it saved me from total destruction. At age 16 I was attending ACOA (Adult Children Of Alcoholics) group meetings, and I read scores of applicable self-help books before I was seventeen.

During my teenage years I was immersed in recovery. Perhaps too much so, but that set the stage for my capacity to keep up with hard emotional recovery work I likely would not have undertaken had it not been for my building endurance. My father, who was obese for most of his life, was immersed in recovery as well. My father was progressive in his recovery work and mastered some very important things.

I regret to say that at age 78 he admits he struggles to defeat his food problems. It's not a surprise to me. There are many key steps that he has been unable to take, such as prayer and meditation. With some people, it's required that they start over and over again on recovery paths until they find a program that works well for them. Employing that level of determination can be difficult for elderly people.

135. Summary and Recap

This book details a comprehensive weight loss program that can be implemented by virtually any individual. This first edition covers quite a bit of ground, addressing a wide variety of interrelated topics. I will make every effort to make whatever stylistic corrections are warranted in future editions. I ask one thing of you: Please seriously consider the book's content and make an effort to do the work. I know you can. You made it this far.

There are a number of concepts that are important to understand when you really want to achieve long-term weight loss and a healthy lifestyle. Some of them may seem abstract or metaphysical in nature. You will be asked to institute a number of positive behavioral changes that seem either foolish or too hard. These things include meditation, writing assignments, dietary improvement, exercise, prayer, and more.

These are the big ones, and each one can seem elusive. There's little excuse in modern times for not knowing how to take the next step forward. This is the information age, and things such as Google and YouTube make additional research and advanced training unbelievably accessible to us all. For example, you could easily search a site like YouTube for instructions on how to begin meditation training.

You and I have a dysfunctional relationship with food, and that relationship needs revisions. In the process of mending the relationship, you need to understand not only what you are doing wrong, but what things have gone wrong in society regarding how food is manufactured, marketed, and distributed.

There is so much that has gone wrong that it's hard to even decide where to begin describing the problems. And the problems are interconnected. Governmental regulating bodies allow food corporations to package and label toxic food. Supermarkets and smaller stores sell such food. People, even those who are well-meaning, raise their children feeding them foods that set them up for lifetime cravings for addictive, self-destructive foods. Other problems include issues with the human psyche, the relationship that we in the modern world have with our planet, and the unique obstacles that each individual encounters while on a path to self-improvement.

I don't like to harp on the negative. But the world around us will still have problematic relationships with food even as we continue to develop. We have to be diligent and stay aware of all of the food distractions that are out there. We must continually be focused on improving our diet and health, even if it causes us some difficulty to do so.

You have to ask yourself: What is the level of my individual desire for self-mastery? I hope that it goes beyond just the desire for weight loss. All human beings should want to reach their higher power. They should want to be the best that they can be.

To succeed, we must learn more about true human nature—that which goes beyond ourselves. Exploring this enables us to understand our deficiencies as a species. One such deficiency—perhaps the foremost one—is that of our child-rearing practices. If other species reared their offspring in ways similar to the ways that we as humans do, they would become extinct.

If we were focused on rearing our children and teaching our peers ways of living that were applicable to our potential for higher consciousness, things would be quite different in the world. We would teach self-love, self-esteem, self-worth, the need for a harmonious relationship with the planet, proper relationships with food, the need for exercise, and the necessity of frequent meditation. These would be revered as the tools that would enable us to survive and flourish.

We human beings need continuous step-by-step training—from the day we were born until the day we die. Of course the most critical time of training is that which takes place during the first 20 years of our lives. This foundational training is crucial—it's the Boot Camp of Life. This training doesn't guarantee that we won't have a variety of struggles, but it will prepare us to deal with them as they arise. I repeat what myriads of others have said: Our training has gone far away from what is right.

The possibilities of what we could create are limitless. But many things that we create do not serve our best interests. One example: We don't need fast food restaurants that serve nothing but incredibly unhealthy, toxic garbage. Such places are a blight on humanity.

We can certainly revel in the advancements (scientific and otherwise) that we've made. But it is a huge mistake to see everything that looks like progress as actually being progress. We have a tendency to marvel at technological advancements without considering the short- and long-term consequences. If that wasn't the case, then we wouldn't have pharmaceutical medications with negative side effects that far outweighed the singular benefits. And there are countless other tragic examples.

We can only overcome our tendency to make such errors by striving to become people that operate at higher levels of consciousness. We need to seek our own happiness in such a way that it doesn't come at the expense of others or at the expense of our planet.

Our environmental errors are prime examples of how our lack of higher consciousness has been problematic for ourselves and others. Our technological advancements in manufacturing have made it so that the creation of massive amounts of garbage harms everyone on the planet.

Broken people were at the forefront of creation of this problem. Greed and self-interest blinded the eyes of those who might have prevented much misery, had they employed social responsibility in the way that they manufactured products and conducted business.

Learning the truth about what happened to us in our childhood is one of life's more painful experiences. We have to uncover difficult events: Doing so brings up painful feelings that we have been avoiding for a lifetime.

There are consequences to keeping these experiences and repressed emotions trapped inside. The consequences of such repression are staring back at us in our adult behaviors and all of the complex character defenses that we created to protect ourselves. Healing is a process of letting these trapped emotions go and then learning new responses.

The work we need to do on ourselves to move forward begins with walking through the dense forest of our past. It's scary for so many reasons, but there is so much hope that comes from braving through the fears of the unknown.

Becoming conscious and awakening yourself is a joyous experience that occurs as we climb higher to the mountain top. Self-knowledge is a gift—not a curse—and this work leads us to it. Unconscious patterns hold us back from being truly and sustainably happy, and we need to overcome them.

In the process of achieving our dietary goals, we will slip up and make mistakes. I call them mistakes, not "moderate living." I don't excuse my mistakes, I forgive them and then move forward. Otherwise, if I make excuses for my mistakes, it keeps a downward spiral going and I won't be able to quit making similar dietary errors. "Moderation" in use of addictive substances, including toxic food products, doesn't work for me.

This book covers a number of the most fundamental aspects of healthy living. Something that will speed up the recovery process tremendously is group therapy or one-on-one therapy. Anyone who is trying to eradicate an addictive cycle should find a group or a therapist that specializes in addictive behavior. The therapist should have some background in 12-step recovery and be well-versed in the foundational aspects of the program that I'm espousing. These foundational aspects include the following entities:

- ► Emotional discovery of past experiences and traumas.
- ► Emotional expression.
- ► Step-by-step behaviors to process emotions and move through them.
- ► Becoming a writer of all aspects of your life.
- ► Diet and overall behavior modification.
- ► Understanding nutrition from the correct perspective.
- ► Behavioral accountability to someone.
- ► Continued education of the nature of self through meditative processes.
- ► Physical exercise and self-care routines that keep the body healthy and keep the mind interested and actively pursuing longevity.
- ► Learning how to meditate/pray/still the mind.

This program espouses the concept that the healed mind pursues longevity. The healed mind is very concentrated and focused on survival.

A key component of survival is good mental health. Mental and physical health must be integrated rather than treated separately. You can't spend seven days a week in analysis and do little or nothing else. Nor can you spend all your time in the gym lifting weights and give no attention to improving your mental health.

Follow as much of this entire program as you can, for as long as it takes to integrate into your life—not in any special order, but rather every day, wherever and whenever you can, activate these tools into your life:

- ▶ Admit that you have a problem (i.e., addiction).
- ▶ Continue your journal: (1) Write an extensive autobiography; (2) Acknowledge admission of your food addiction problem(s) and associated behaviors; (3) Write out every step required to be restored to optimal thinking and happiness free from the suffering created in your mind, and (4) Write out every addiction you have and become ready to surrender doing any of them.
- ▶ Create the following lists: (1) People you have harmed; (2) People who have harmed you; (3) Things you love; (4) Things you dislike; (5) Wish list; and (6) A list of solutions.
- ▶ Childhood discovery writings: Write about your childhood traumas and discover the disturbances in your upbringing.
- ▶ Share these lists and key writings with another person.
- ▶ Change or become willing to change your diet in the following ways: (1) Eliminate processed foods; (2) Do not eat late at night; (3) Reduce the amount of protein in general, especially animal protein; (4) Consider going 100% plant-based; (5) Do not follow fad diets; (6) Fall in love with the good sugar in fruit and starchy vegetables; (7) Make the carbohydrates your primary source of fuel, i.e., the carbohydrates from fruits and vegetables; (8) Drink clean water; (9) Pay attention to how you combine foods together; (10) Eliminate dairy food from cows; and (11) Eliminate alcohol and tobacco.
- ▶ Practice meditation.

- ► Use breathing exercises throughout the day to maintain excellent oxygen levels to the brain for clarity and focus.
- ► Pray to a higher power.
- ► Be of service to others. Especially as it pertains to the specific item we are trying to improve in ourselves. In other words, help others with the same needs to facilitate alleviating our own problems.
- ► Exercise. Get passionate about good movement. Use your body.
- ► Play close attention to the way you feel throughout each day. Have a plan for what to do in different situations when you feel compelled to eat to change our emotions.
- ► Maintenance: Repeat the items on this list of activities daily throughout life.

136. My Top 30 Positive Health and Lifestyle Changes/Behaviors

Following is a list of 30 important items in the overall addiction recovery program that I follow.

1. Breathe clean air (a primary nutrient): In addition to doing that, you should do simple breathing exercises daily, speak out against air pollution, and do what you can to ensure that future generations have clean air to breathe as well.

2. Drink a lot of clean water every day: It's crucial that you do so, and you must ensure that it's clean,

whether you get it from a stream in a pristine environment, get high quality bottled water, or filter your own home water system.

3. Eliminate all processed foods from your diet: Getting toxic food components and additives out of your system will yield health benefits for you very quickly.

4. Get plenty of total body exercise: Movement is required every day. Make sure that you practice exercises that keep you flexible and strong, and that increase your balance, your focus, and your body's ability to learn.

5. Stop smoking cigarettes or inhaling marijuana smoke into your lungs: Both of those things are highly toxic.

6. Go to the bathroom frequently: Eliminate your waste, as being backed up causes not only physical problems but mental and emotional problems as well.

7. Reduce your intake of animal protein or eliminate it completely: You will become a mobile, biologically efficient creature if you are eating the foods that you are biologically compatible with—specifically, plant-based foods.

8. Get plenty of rest: Both the mind and body conduct healing and restorative functions during such times.

9. Eliminate cow's milk and dairy products: If you feel the desperate need to include cheese in your diet, use the raw cheeses from goats and sheep, although total abstinence from dairy products is preferable.

10. Eliminate alcohol, drugs, and similar substances: They are all toxic and detrimental to your health and wellness in many ways.

11. Practice meditation: It will help you get control over thoughts that continually distract your mind, and will also contribute considerably to your physical and mental health.

12. Face up to and deal with all of your emotions: Doing so is a long-term endeavor that will enable you to overcome painful, persistent setbacks that interfere tremendously with health, wellness, happiness, productivity, and peace of mind.

13. Practice honesty in everything that you do: In addition to communicating the essence of your true self, you grow tremendously as a person when you are honest. You foster courage, display maturity, build interpersonal connections, and clear out "emotional baggage" in such a way that it builds your self-image.

14. Apologize often: Almost every day of our lives we have an opportunity to express an apology to someone. It's an act that shows strength of character and courage on our part, and it gives us a good reason to respect ourselves.

15. Don't overeat: It goes without saying that the consequences of overeating are extremely detrimental in quite a number of ways to your overall quality of life.

16. Don't eat late at night: Human chemistry is designed to clean up and repair the body after sunset, and eating at night requires that the body engages in digestion, which subsequently interferes with its needed focus on bodily cleanup and repair.

17. Combine foods properly: In any single meal, make sure to eat foods that are compatible with each other so that effective digestion will occur.

18. Maintain your teeth. Good oral hygiene is important not just to have teeth to chew with, but to avoid a variety of diseases related both to the mouth and to digestion.

19. Keep your body clean: You can prevent illness and infections from viruses and bacteria by practicing good hygiene at all times.

20. Take plant-based dietary supplements: High-quality, high-potency, plant-based supplements will stimulate your body in a beautiful way provided that you don't use them indiscriminately or in excess.

21. Experience joy and laughter: Doing so benefits your organs and immune system, increases serotonin and endorphins in the brain, and decreases stress hormones in the body.

22. Maintain and preserve important relationships with other people, with animals, and with nature: Human beings are relational creatures who can only function at their optimum levels when they relate effectively to all entities that touch their lives.

23. Believe in something: A sense of purpose that drives positive actions on a person's part stimulates good mind and body functionality in a wide variety of ways.

24. Focus on things that you are grateful for daily: Studies have shown that gratitude is associated with good cardiovascular health, counteracting depression, improved sleep, lessening of aches and pains, happiness, and improved relationships.

25. Keep your living space clean: Not only does cleanliness ensure less spread of germs, but it creates an environment where you can be less stressed, more focused, and more productive in all of your activities.

26. Show respect to your teachers: You can "give credit where credit's due" by showing appreciation for and to those who have enhanced your life by imparting their helpful knowledge to you.

27. Avoid these particular foods: All fried items, pork, and ocean and freshwater bottom-feeding creatures are among the worst foods for your overall health.

28. Show compassion: The many benefits of compassion that have been proven through studies include reduction of stress, decreased mental instability, heightened social awareness, and increased happiness.

29. Practice forgiveness: Also proven through studies, acts of forgiveness significantly enhance good health by reducing anxiety, pain, blood pressure, stress, and depression, and by improving cholesterol levels, sleep, happiness, and overall peace of mind.

30. Keep a journal: Communicating in writing clarifies things for you and helps bring intangible thought concepts into realities that you can take action on. You become a more efficient, productive, and emotionally healthy individual when you do so.

137. Maintenance: We Need Daily Tune-Ups

You are a high performance race car, not a dump truck. Consider your emotional and psychological work to be processes that keep your mind and body in top working order. Also realize that in order to operate and run smoothly, you need to adhere to a program like this perpetually. The way to do that is to continue to do this type of work throughout all of the times of your life, whether experiencing happiness or horror.

If you think you are enlightened, you probably are. However, something can pull you off center: A mosquito bite, a pandemic, the death of a loved one, our children, our lovers, spouses, bosses, presidents, taxes, and so on. There's a list a mile long of the things and events that can distract you from mental stillness. The adjustment back to center is as easy as you make it. It is possible to return to an emotional equilibrium as you do maintenance work in between the serious and difficult moments of your life.

Continue to work to monitor your emotions and state of mind every day by writing in your calendar or your journal. Don't get complacent when you feel happy. Happiness is a motivator to dig deeper and bolster your protective wall that will later protect you from the possibility of a relapse.

138. Confusement

I realize from all the years of work on myself and all of the observations that I've made in the people that I was fortunate to help in 12-step recovery, there are times when facing intellectual challenges and solving problems seems impossible.

There are times when you will feel like a five-year-old child lost at a supermarket. You won't even be able to look at the words in this book. You might take this book and hide it underneath other books, or forget it at a coffee shop, or give it away, because you feel that there's too much information, too many requirements, and a lot of what I call "confusement."

To alleviate this problem, I've formatted the book in a way that I hope you'll find helpful. The numbered section titles refer to specific problems and solutions to things that you may be struggling with. You can refer to a particular section to help you with a particular negative feeling that you might be struggling with, or to review some information about a particular dietary issue that arises at any given time. And in casual reading it may be easier to read the book in sections as well.

Pick up the book at random times and just open it and read any section. Then close your eyes, put the book down and say, "OK, what I just read, did any of it resonate for me? Did it leave any questions?"

It's unlikely that you'll find a good philosophical process or really solid lifelong message that you could pick up in a few hours. Much of the content of the book consists of things that must be considered for a very long time before they soak in.

Remember that there's a big part of you that doesn't want to change. It's a mysterious part of me that I look for all the time and try to figure out what that side of me needs. But most of the time I just have to take positive action. And books like these give me plenty of that to do. If I'm doing something from a good book that I really can relate to, I'm confident that I'm doing the work.

139. Self-Acceptance: When You Have It, You Know You Are Getting Well

Self-acceptance is crucial right from the beginning. You have to tell yourself that you are not just your body: You're so many other things. You can start off with exercises of looking in the mirror and saying thank you to your body for all of the hard work that it does for you. I know that sounds really corny but it's a reversal of the type of things that you tell yourself 16 hours of the day.

Positive messages to yourself over time will have a positive impact. It's phenomenal how something so silly works so effectively. No matter what body type you are, you are wonderful and you are deserving of many gifts and many blessings. As much time as you spend focusing on the negative attributes of yourself, spend 10 times the same amount pleasing yourself.

But don't do it in an outrageous and braggadocious kind of way. By doing that, you will turn into an asshole. The concept is that you should quietly, by yourself, and remind yourself of the nice things that you do and the things that make you good.

Say them out loud and write them on paper so that they materialize and have power. By materializing, I mean that if you keep saying those things you will eventually truly believe them. And then they will affect every fiber of your physical body—every cell.

140. Recovering From Mistakes and Relapses

In the process of achieving your diet goals, you will slip up and make mistakes. Call them mistakes, not "moderate living." Otherwise, it will keep a downward spiral going and you won't be able to quit making your dietary errors. "Moderation" in use of addictive substances, including toxic food products, doesn't work.

I really appreciate you for taking this journey—you're amazing. You are special, and you are a pure light behind that body. The body does matter, and keeping it healthy and right is one the many tests and challenges for all living creatures.

I hope that you find the things that make you happy and that you share that happiness with the world. Don't let the negativity of the outside or inside world influence you and distract you. Instead, let any negativity that you have inside find its way to your writing and forever set it free.

Thank you for reading this book, and I hope that it will continue to lead you into a great new lifestyle that encompasses good health and higher consciousness.

141. Inspiration to Continue Getting Better

This is a lengthy book, and I know it will take time for you to absorb the information and put it into action. I encourage you to do the same thing I did when I was in Alcoholics Anonymous beginning at age 15. Instinctively, I felt the best thing to do was to keep the Big Book close at hand and read it cover to cover four times. I memorized certain chapters. Slowly but surely, the information began to materialize in my head.

At times my attention would drift, and to some degree I felt that the information in the book didn't have the level of direct instruction that I desired. This is the main reason that I've put so much content into this book. I want to cover as much as I can and give you all of the information and tools that you will need.

I have seen and interacted with a huge number of people who struggled terribly with food addictions, anxiety problems, and addictions to adrenaline, alcohol, and drugs who succeeded at becoming normalized by following this type of program.

I know that being able to take the direction that this book offers will require tremendous courage and patience. You have both. You will succeed in this effort. Keep telling yourself that. This is exactly the same power that a fighter gets before he or she goes into the ring. They tell themselves backstage while warming up, "I'm going to win, I'm going to win, I'm going to win," and they visualize themselves winning. They see themselves raising their hand up in victory. They see themselves in exactly the successful position they want to be in. That has an enormous, enormous impact on their wills.

Follow in the footsteps of those men and women. Don't let your negative voice take over and tell you that this is foolish, or you'll never make it, or that there's no point in trying. That thinking does not serve you anymore. Let go of it!

From now on write only positive words down on the pages of your journal. When you're talking about the things that happened to you in the past, you may need to write about certain unpleasant, negative things. But when you're talking about the things that are happening to you right now and your thoughts and actions going forward, talk about them in the most positive way that you can.

You can be a great coach to yourself. Take a lot of pride and gratitude in the fact that you completed this book. You're now going to do the work, and step by step you are going to get better!

I sincerely hope to see you as we both move along on our mutual paths to happiness and peace of mind.

Please visit www.goodsugardiet.com for support pages on this program. Included are free recipes and daily meal suggestions.

Please email questions, comments, and suggestions for possible integration into future editions of this program: info@goodsugar.life

About the Author

Marcus Antebi founded a health and wellness platform in New York called Juice Press. He has been writing about diet, general health, fitness, and recovery for 20 years.

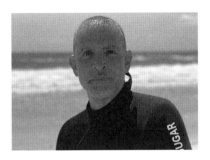

> "The essence of this book was taught to me throughout my life. The ingredients were never mine. All I did was mix them and add my own flavors. I borrowed good philosophy from every wellspring that I know of that contains timeless human knowledge. Therefore, all of the thoughts expressed in this work would be pointless if they weren't intended to be given back to all of humanity. I checked with my neighbor, my sponsor, two shamans, my wife, my food guru, my yoga teacher, and my conscience, and all of those sources verified that this work is clear and compassionate."
>
> **—MARCUS ANTEBI**
> *Founder, Author, Athlete, and other things.*